Fix-It and Forget-It®
INSTANT POT
DIABETES
COOKBOOK

127 SUPER EASY HEALTHY RECIPES

HOPE COMERFORD

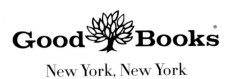

Good Books

New York, New York

Table of Contents

Welcome to *Fix-It and Forget-It Instant Pot Diabetes Cookbook* ⚘ 1

What Is an Instant Pot? ⚘ 1

Getting Started with Your Instant Pot ⚘ 1

Instant Pot Tips and Tricks and Other Things You May Not Know ⚘ 5

Calculating the Nutritional Analysis ⚘ 6

Tips for Healthier, Happier Eating ⚘ 7

How to Plan Healthy Meals ⚘ 7

Learning Portion Control ⚘ 8

Frequently Asked Questions About Diabetes and Food ⚘ 9

Breakfast ⚘ 13

Appetizers & Snacks ⚘ 37

Soups, Stews, Chilies & Chowders ⚘ 63

Main Dishes ⚘ 117

Side Dishes & Vegetables ⚘ 191

Desserts ⚘ 225

Metric Equivalent Measurements ⚘ 252

Recipe and Ingredient Index ⚘ 253

About the Author ⚘ 260

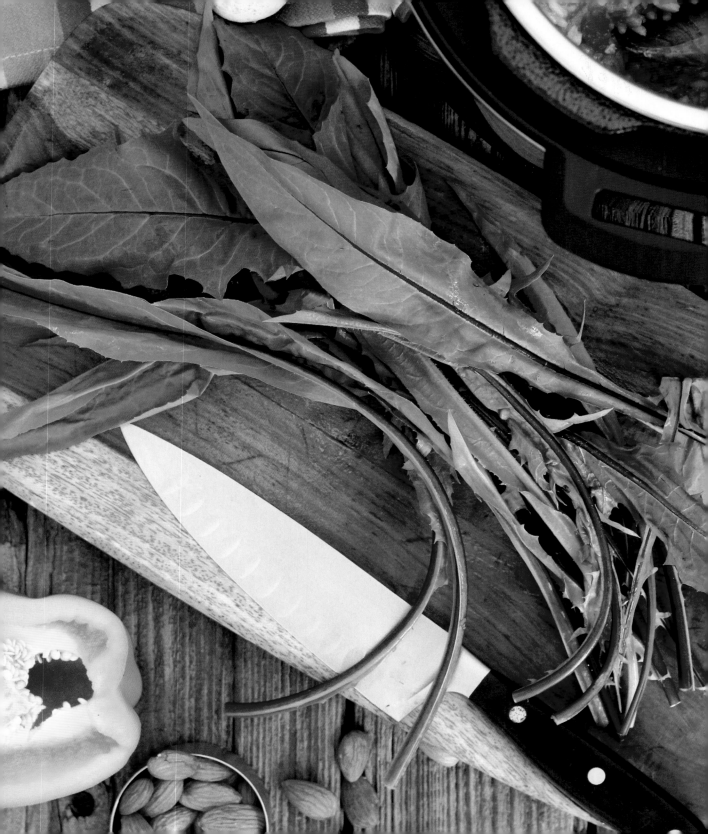

Welcome to *Fix-It and Forget-It Instant Pot Diabetes Cookbook*

There is a lot of worry that comes with being on any kind of a special diet. We're happy to have the brand new *Fix-It and Forget-It Instant Pot Diabetes Cookbook* available to you with 127 recipes you know will fit your dietary restrictions. When you're diabetic, it's important to manage your calorie, carb, fat, and sodium counts. That's why we've put together these recipes, each with nutritional information included, so you and your loved ones can enjoy your meals without the guesswork. Each recipe is followed by its Exchange List Values, listing carbs, fats, starches, etc. and the Basic Nutritional Values as well.

You'll find this cookbook to be full of easy recipes everyday home cooks can tackle with their Instant Pot. If you're new to Instant-Potting, just getting your feet wet, or are a total newbie, fear not! This cookbook has you covered! Even if you're a seasoned Instant-Potter, I'm sure you'll be thrilled to find some new recipes to add to your rotation of Instant Pot recipes.

Fix-It and Forget-It has always brought you recipes for your slow-cooker you can make with confidence and ease. We are thrilled to be bringing you something new! We think you're going to love using your Instant Pot and can't wait for you to get started!

What Is an Instant Pot?

In short, an Instant Pot is a digital pressure cooker that also has multiple other functions. Not only can it be used as a pressure cooker, but depending on which model Instant Pot you have, you can set it to do things like sauté, cook rice, multigrains, porridge, soup/stew, beans/chili, porridge, meat, poultry, cake, eggs, yogurt, steam, slow cook or even set it manually. Because the Instant Pot has so many functions, it takes away the need for multiple appliances on your counter and allows you to use fewer pots and pans.

Getting Started With Your Instant Pot

Get to Know Your Instant Pot . . .

The very first thing most Instant Pot owners do is called the water test. It helps you get to know your Instant Pot a bit, familiarizes you with it, and might even take a bit of your apprehension away (because if you're anything like me, I was scared to death to use it!).

Step 1: Plug in your Instant Pot. This may seem obvious to some, but when we're nervous about using a new appliance, sometimes we forget things like this.

Step 2: Make sure the inner pot is inserted in the cooker. You should NEVER attempt to cook anything in your device without the inner pot, or you will ruin your Instant Pot. Food should never come into contact with the actual housing unit.

Step 3: The inner pot has lines for each cup (how convenient, right?!) Fill the inner pot with water until it reaches the 3-cup line.

Step 4: Check the sealing ring to be sure it's secure and in place. You should not be able to move it around. If it's not in place properly, you may experience issues with the pot letting out a lot of steam while cooking, or not coming to pressure.

Step 5: Seal the lid. There is an arrow on the lid between and "open" and "close." There is also an arrow on the top of the base of the Instant Pot between a picture of a locked lock and an unlocked lock. Line those arrows up, then turn the lid toward the picture of the lock (left). You will hear a noise that will indicate the lid is locked. If you do not hear a noise, it's not locked. Try it again.

Step 6: ALWAYS check to see if the steam valve on top of the lid is turned to "sealing." If it's not on "sealing" and is on "venting," it will not be able to come to pressure.

Step 7: Press the "Steam" button and use the +/- arrow to set it to 2 minutes. Once it's at the desired time, you don't need to press anything else. In a few seconds, the Instant Pot will begin all on its own. For those of us with digital slow cookers, we have a tendency to look for the "start" button, but there isn't one on the Instant Pot.

Step 8: Now you wait for the "magic" to happen! The "cooking" will begin once the device comes to pressure. This can take anywhere from 5 to 30 minutes I've found in my experience. Then, you will see the countdown happen (from the time you set it at). After that, the Instant Pot will beep, which means your meal is done!

Step 9: Your Instant Pot will now automatically switch to "warm" and begin a count of how many minutes it's been on warm. The next part is where you either wait for the NPR, or natural pressure release (meaning the pressure releases all on its own) or you do what's called a QR, or quick release (meaning, you manually release the pressure). Which method you choose depends on what you're cooking, but in this case, you can choose either since it's just water. For NPR, you will wait for the lever to move all the way back over to "venting" and watch the pinion (float valve) next to the lever. It will be flush with the lid when at full pressure and will drop when the pressure is done releasing. If you choose QR, be very careful not to have your hands over the vent as the steam is very hot and you can burn yourself.

Making a Foil Sling
In many recipes in this book, you'll see instructions to make a foil sling. To do so, cut a length of aluminum foil that's about 20 inches long. Fold it into thirds, lengthwise. Place it beneath the inner pot. This makes it easy to remove the inner pot later without spilling its contents!

The Three Most Important Buttons You Need to Know About . . .

You will find the majority of recipes will use the following three buttons:

Manual/Pressure Cook: Some older models tend to say "Manual" and the newer models seem to say "Pressure Cook." They mean the same thing. From here, you use the +/- button to change the cook time. After several seconds, the Instant Pot will begin its process. The exact name of this button will vary on your model of Instant Pot.

Sauté: Many recipes will have you sauté vegetables, or brown meat before beginning the pressure cooking process. For this setting, you will not use the lid of the Instant Pot.

Keep Warm/Cancel: This may just be the most important button on the Instant Pot. When you forget to use the +/- buttons to change the time for a recipe, or you press a wrong button, you can hit "Keep Warm/Cancel" and it will turn your Instant Pot off for you.

What Do All the Buttons Do . . .

With so many buttons, it's hard to remember what each one does or means. You can use this as a quick guide in a pinch.

Soup/Broth. This button cooks at high pressure for 30 minutes. It can be adjusted using the +/- buttons to cook more for 40 minutes, or less for 20 minutes.

Meat/Stew. This button cooks at high pressure for 35 minutes. It can be adjusted using the +/- buttons to cook more for 45 minutes, or less for 20 minutes.

Bean/Chili. This button cooks at high pressure for 30 minutes. It can be adjusted using the +/- buttons to cook more for 40 minutes, or less for 25 minutes.

Poultry. This button cooks at high pressure for 15 minutes. It can be adjusted using the +/- buttons to cook more for 30 minutes, or less for 5 minutes.

Rice. This button cooks at low pressure and is the only fully automatic program. It is for cooking white rice and will automatically adjust the cooking time depending on the amount of water and rice in the cooking pot.

Multigrain. This button cooks at high pressure for 40 minutes. It can be adjusted using the +/- buttons to cook more for 45 minutes of warm water soaking time and 60 minutes pressure-cooking time, or less for 20 minutes.

Porridge. This button cooks at high pressure for 20 minutes. It can be adjusted using the +/- buttons to cook more for 30 minutes, or less for 15 minutes.

Steam. This button cooks at high pressure for 10 minutes. It can be adjusted using the +/- buttons to cook more for 15 minutes, or less for 3 minutes. Always use a rack or steamer basket with this function because it heats at full power continuously while it's coming to pressure and you do not want food in direct contact with the bottom of the pressure cooking pot or it will burn. Once it reaches pressure, the steam button regulates pressure by cycling on and off, similar to the other pressure buttons.

Less | Normal | More. Adjust between the *Less | Normal | More* settings by pressing the same cooking function button repeatedly until you get to the desired setting. (Older versions use the *Adjust* button.)

+/- Buttons. Adjust the cook time up [+] or down [-]. (On newer models, you can also press and hold [-] or [+] for 3 seconds to turn sound OFF or ON.)

Cake. This button cooks at high pressure for 30 minutes. It can be adjusted using the +/- buttons to cook more for 40 minutes, or less for 25 minutes.

Egg. This button cooks at high pressure for 5 minutes. It can be adjusted using the +/- buttons to cook more for 6 minutes, or less for 4 minutes.

Instant Pot Tips and Tricks and Other Things You May Not Know

- Never attempt to cook directly in the Instant Pot without the Inner Pot!
- Once you set the time, you can walk away. It will show the time you set it to, then will change to the word "on" while the pressure builds. Once the Instant Pot has come to pressure, you will once again see the time you set it for. It will count down from there.
- Always make sure your sealing ring is securely in place. Many people find it useful to have a sealing ring for sweet dishes and one for savory dishes. If it shows signs of wear or tear, it needs to be replaced.
- Have a sealing ring for savory recipes and a separate sealing ring for sweet recipes. Many people report of their desserts tasting like a roast (or another savory food) if they try to use the same sealing ring for all recipes.
- The stainless steel rack (trivet) your Instant Pot comes with can used to keep food from being completely submerged in liquid, like baked potatoes or ground beef. It can also be used to set another pot on, for pot-in-pot cooking.
- If you use warm or hot liquid instead of cold liquid, you may need to adjust the cooking time, or your food may not come out done.
- Always double-check to see that the valve on the lid is set to "sealing" and not "venting" when you first lock the lid. This will save you from your Instant Pot not coming to pressure.
- Use Natural Pressure Release for tougher cuts of meat, recipes with high starch (like rice or grains) and recipes with a high volume of liquid. This means you let the Instant Pot naturally release pressure. The little bobbin will fall once pressure is released completely.
- Use quick release for more delicate cuts of meat and vegetables–like seafood, chicken breasts, and steaming vegetables. This means you manually turn the vent (being careful not to put your hand over the vent!) to release the pressure. The little bobbin will fall once pressure is released completely.
- Make sure there is a clear pathway for the steam to release. The last thing you want is to ruin the bottom of your cupboards with all that steam.
- You MUST use liquid in your Instant Pot. The MINIMUM amount of liquid you should have in your inner pot is ½ cup, however, most recipes work best with at least 1 cup.
- Do NOT overfill your Instant Pot! It should only be ½ full for rice or beans (food that expands greatly when cooked) or ⅔ of the way full for most everything else. Do not fill it to the max filled line.

- In this book, the Cooking Time DOES NOT take into account the amount of time it will take your Instant Pot to come to pressure, or the amount of time it will take the instant pot to release pressure. Be aware of this when choosing a recipe to make.
- If your Instant Pot is not coming to pressure, it's usually because the sealing ring is not on properly, or the vent is not set to "sealing."
- The more liquid, or the colder the ingredients, the longer it will take for the Instant Pot to come to pressure.
- Always make sure that the Instant Pot is dry before inserting the inner pot, and make sure the inner pot is dry before inserting it into the Instant Pot.
- Doubling a recipe does not change the cook time, but instead it will take longer to come up to pressure.
- You do not always need to double the liquid when doubling a recipe. Depending on what you're making, more liquid may make your food too watery. Use your best judgment.
- When using the Slow Cook function, use the following chart:

Slow Cooker	Instant Pot
Warm	Less or Low
Low	Normal or Medium
High	More or High

Calculating the Nutritional Analysis

If the number of servings is given as a range, we used the higher number to do the nutritional analyses calculations.

The nutritional analysis for each recipe includes all ingredients except those labeled "optional," those listed as "to taste," or those calling for a "dash." If an ingredient is listed with a second choice, the first choice was used in the analysis. If a range is given for the amount of an ingredient, the first number was used. Foods listed as "serve with" at the end of a recipe, or accompanying foods listed without an amount, were not included in the recipe's analysis. In recipes calling for cooked rice, pasta, or other grains, the analysis is based on the starch being prepared without added salt or fat, unless indicated otherwise in the recipe. Please note, too, that the nutritional analyses do not cover the ingredients included in the Tips and Variations which accompany some of the recipes.

The analyses were done assuming that meats were trimmed of all visible fat, and that skin was removed from poultry, before being cooked.

Tips for Healthier, Happier Eating

How to Plan Healthy Meals

Healthy meal planning is an important part of diabetes care. If you have diabetes, you should have a meal plan specifying what, when, and how much you should eat. Work with a registered dietitian to create a meal plan that is right for you. A typical meal plan covers your meals and snacks and includes a variety of foods. Here are some popular meal-planning tools:

1. **An exchange list** is a list of foods that are grouped together because they share similar carbohydrate, protein, and fat content. Any food on an exchange list may be substituted for any other food on the same list. A meal plan that uses exchange lists will tell you the number of exchanges (or food choices) you can eat at each meal or snack. You then choose the foods that add up to those exchanges.

2. **Carbohydrate counting** is useful because carbohydrates are the main nutrient in food that affects blood glucose. When you count carbohydrates, you simply count up the carbohydrates in the foods you eat, which helps you manage your blood glucose levels. To find the carbohydrate content of a food, check the Nutrition Facts label on foods or ask your dietitian for help. Carbohydrate counting is especially helpful for people with diabetes who take insulin to help manage their blood glucose.

3. **The Create Your Plate method** helps people with diabetes put together meals with evenly distributed carbohydrate content and correct portion sizes. This is one of the easiest meal-planning options because it does not require any special tools—all you need is a plate. Fill half of your plate with non-starchy vegetables, such as spinach, carrots, cabbage, green beans, or broccoli. Fill one-quarter of the plate with starchy foods, such as rice, pasta, beans, or peas. Fill the final quarter of your plate with meat or a meat substitute, such as cheese with less than 3 grams of fat per ounce, cottage cheese, or egg substitute. For a balanced meal, add a serving of low-fat or nonfat milk and a serving of fruit.

No matter which tool you use to plan your meals, having a meal plan in place can help you manage your blood glucose levels, improve your cholesterol levels, and maintain a healthy blood pressure and a healthy weight. When you're able to do that, you're helping to control—or avoid—diabetes.

Learning Portion Control

Portion control is an important part of healthier eating. Weighing and measuring your foods helps familiarize yourself with reasonable portions and can make a difference of several hundred calories each day. You want to frequently weigh and measure your foods when you begin following a healthy eating plan. The more you practice weighing and measuring, the easier it will become to accurately estimate portion sizes.

You'll want to have certain portion-control tools on hand when you're weighing and measuring your foods. Remember, the teaspoons and tablespoons in your silverware set won't give you exact measurements. Here's what goes into your portion-control toolbox:

- Measuring spoons for ½ teaspoon, 1 teaspoon, ½ tablespoon, and 1 tablespoon
- A see-through 1-cup measuring cup with markings at ¼, ⅓, ½, ⅔, and ¾ cup
- Measuring cups for dry ingredients, including ¼, ⅓, ½, and 1 cup.

You may already have most of these in your kitchen. Keep them on your counter—you are more likely to use these tools if you can see them. Get an inexpensive food scale for foods that are measured in ounces, such as fresh produce, baked goods, meats, and cheese. When you're weighing meat, poultry, and seafood, keep in mind that you will need more than 3 ounces of raw meat to produce a 3-ounce portion of cooked meat. For example, it takes 4 ounces of raw, boneless meat—or 5 ounces of raw meat with the bone—to produce 3 cooked ounces. About 4½ ounces of raw chicken (with the bone and skin) yields 3 ounces cooked. Remember to remove the skin from the chicken before eating it.

There are other easy ways to control your portions at home in addition to weighing and measuring:

- Eat on smaller plates and bowls so that small portions look normal, not skimpy.
- Use a measuring cup to serve food to easily determine how much you're serving and eating.
- Measure your drinking glasses and bowls, so you know how much you're drinking or eating when you fill them.
- Avoid serving your meals family-style because leaving large serving dishes on the table can lead to second helpings and overeating.
- Keep portion sizes in mind while shopping. When you buy meat, fish, or poultry, purchase only what you need for your meal.

When you're away from home, your eyes and hands become your portion-control tools. You can use your hand to estimate teaspoons, tablespoons, ounces, and cups. The tip of your thumb is about 1 teaspoon; your whole thumb equals roughly 1 tablespoon. Two fingers lengthwise are about an ounce, and 3 ounces is about the size of a palm. You can use your fist to measure in cups. A tight fist is about half a cup, whereas a loose fist or cupped hand is closer to a cup.

These guidelines are true for most women's hands, but some men's hands are much larger.

The palm of a man's hand is often the equivalent of about 5 ounces. Check the size of your hand in relation to various portions.

Remember that the more you weigh and measure your foods at home, the easier it will be to estimate portions on the road.

Controlling your portions when you eat at a restaurant can be difficult. Try to stay away from menu items with portion descriptors that are large, such as "giant," "supreme," "extra-large," "double," "triple," "king-size," and "super." Don't fall for deals in which the "value" is to serve you more food so that you can save money. Avoid all-you-can-eat restaurants and buffets.

You can split, share, or mix and match menu items to get what you want to eat in the correct portions. If you know that the portions you'll be served will be too large, ask for a take-home container when you place your order and put half of your food away before you start eating.

Gradually, as you become better at portion control, you can weigh and measure your foods less frequently. If you feel like you are correctly estimating your portions, just weigh and measure once a week, or even once a month, to check that your portions are still accurate. A good habit to get into is to "calibrate" your portion-control memory at least once a month, so you don't start underestimating your portion sizes. Always weigh and measure new foods and foods that you tend to underestimate.

Frequently Asked Questions about Diabetes and Food

1. *Do people with diabetes have to eat a special diet?*
No, they should eat the same foods that are healthy for everyone—whole grains, vegetables, fruit, and small portions of lean meat. Like everyone else, people with diabetes should eat breakfast, lunch, and dinner and not put off eating until dinnertime. By then, you are ravenous and will eat too much. This sends blood sugar levels soaring in people with diabetes and doesn't allow them to feel hungry for breakfast the next morning.

2. *Can people with diabetes eat sugar?*
Yes, they can. Sugar is just another carbohydrate to the body. All carbohydrates, whether they come from dessert, breads, or carrots, raise blood sugar. An equal serving of brownie and of baked

potato raise your blood sugar the same amount. If you know that a rise in blood sugar is coming, it is wise to focus on the size of the serving. The question of "how much sugar is too much?" has to be answered by each one of us. No one who wants to be healthy eats a lot of sugar.

3. What natural substances are good sugar substitutes? Are artificial sweeteners safe for people with diabetes?
Honey, agave nectar, maple syrup, brown sugar, and white sugar all contain about the same amount of calories and have a similar effect on your blood glucose levels. All of these sweeteners are a source of carbohydrates and will raise blood glucose quickly.

If you have diabetes, you can use these sweeteners sparingly if you work them into your meal plan. Be aware of portion sizes and the carbohydrate content of each sweetener:

- 1 tablespoon honey = about 64 calories, 17 grams of carbohydrate
- 1 tablespoon brown sugar = about 52 calories, 13 grams of carbohydrate
- 1 tablespoon white sugar = about 48 calories, 13 grams of carbohydrate
- 1 tablespoon agave nectar = about 45 calories, 12 grams of carbohydrate
- 1 tablespoon maple syrup = about 52 calories, 13 grams of carbohydrate
- 1 packet of artificial sweetener = about 4 calories, <1 gram of carbohydrate

Artificial sweeteners are a low-calorie, low-carb option. Because they are chemically modified to be sweeter than regular sugar, only a small amount is needed to sweeten foods and drinks. There are several different artificial sweeteners available under various brand names: stevia, aspartame, acesulfame-K, saccharin, or sucralose. With the direction of your health care provider, these may be safe options for people with diabetes when used in moderate amounts.

4. How many grams of carbohydrates should someone with diabetes eat per day? How many at each meal?
This is a very common question. About 45–60 grams of carbohydrates per meal is a good starting point when you are carb-counting. If you follow that recommendation, you will be eating a total of 135–180 grams of carbohydrates per day. However, some people may need more, and some may need less. Talk with your health care team to create an individualized meal plan to help you meet your health goals.

5. What types of fruit can I eat? Is canned or fresh fruit better for people with diabetes?
You can eat any type of fruit if you work it into your meal plan. Fruits are loaded with vitamins, minerals, and fiber. Fresh, canned, or frozen fruit without added sugars are all good

options. You get a similar amount of nutrients from each. When you buy canned fruit, be sure the fruit has been canned in water or juice—not in syrup.

Fruit is nutritious, but it is not a "free food." The following portions have about 15 grams of carbohydrates:

- 1 small piece of whole fruit such as a small apple, small orange, or kiwifruit
- ½ cup of frozen or canned fruit
- ¾–1 cup of fresh berries or melon
- ⅓–½ cup 100% no-sugar-added fruit juice
- 2 tablespoons of dried fruit

6. Besides meat, what can I eat to make sure I get enough protein?

There are many protein sources. Proteins that are low in saturated and trans fats are the best options. Choose lean sources of protein like these:

- Eggs, egg whites, and egg substitutes
- Vegetarian proteins: beans, soy products, veggie burgers, nuts, and seeds
- Low-fat or nonfat dairy products
- Fish and shellfish
- Poultry without the skin
- Cheeses with 3 grams of fat or less per ounce
- When you do eat meat, choose lean cuts

People with diabetes can follow a vegetarian or vegan diet. Plant-based diets that include some animal products like eggs and milk can be a healthy option. However, animal products are not necessary. A mix of soy products, vegetables, fruits, beans, and whole grains provides plenty of protein and nutrients.

7. Why should I eat whole grains instead of refined grains?

Even a food made with 100% whole wheat flour will raise your blood glucose levels. All grains—whole or not—affect blood glucose because they contain carbohydrates. However, you shouldn't completely avoid starchy foods. People with diabetes need some carbohydrates in their diet.

Whole grains are a healthy starch option because they contain fiber, vitamins, and minerals. Choose whole wheat or whole grain foods over those made with refined grains, but watch your portion sizes.

8. *Can people with diabetes eat potatoes and sweet potatoes?*

Yes! Starchy vegetables are healthy sources of carbohydrates. They also provide you with important nutrients like potassium, fiber, and vitamin C. You can include them in your meal plan as part of a balanced meal. Just pay attention to portion sizes and avoid unhealthy toppings. If you are carb-counting, remember that there are about 15 grams of carbohydrates in:

- ½ cup of mashed potatoes
- ½ cup of boiled potatoes
- ¼ of a large baked potato with the skin

9. *Without salt and fat, food tastes bland. What can I do?*

When you are preparing healthy foods, try to limit added fats and extra salt. Look for recipes that use herbs (fresh or dried) and spices for flavor instead. There are many spice blends available in the baking aisle at the grocery store—choose salt-free blends. Other healthy ways to flavor your foods include:

- Squeezing lemon or lime juice on vegetables, fish, rice, or pasta
- Using onion and garlic to flavor dishes
- Baking meats with sugar-free barbecue sauce or any low-fat marinade
- Adding low-fat, low-calorie condiments, such as mustard, salsa, balsamic vinegar, or hot sauce

10. *Are gluten-free products okay for people with diabetes to eat?*

About 1% of the total population has celiac disease, which is an allergy to gluten—a protein found in wheat, rye, and barley. About 10% of people with type 1 diabetes also have celiac disease. People with celiac disease or gluten intolerance should follow a gluten-free diet.

However, unless you have one of these conditions, following a gluten-free diet is unnecessary and can make meal planning more difficult. Gluten-free products may contain more grams of carbohydrates per serving than regular products. For example, gluten-free bread can have twice as many grams of carbohydrates as whole wheat bread. You can use gluten-free products and recipes, but just be sure to check the carbohydrate content and calories.

Breakfast

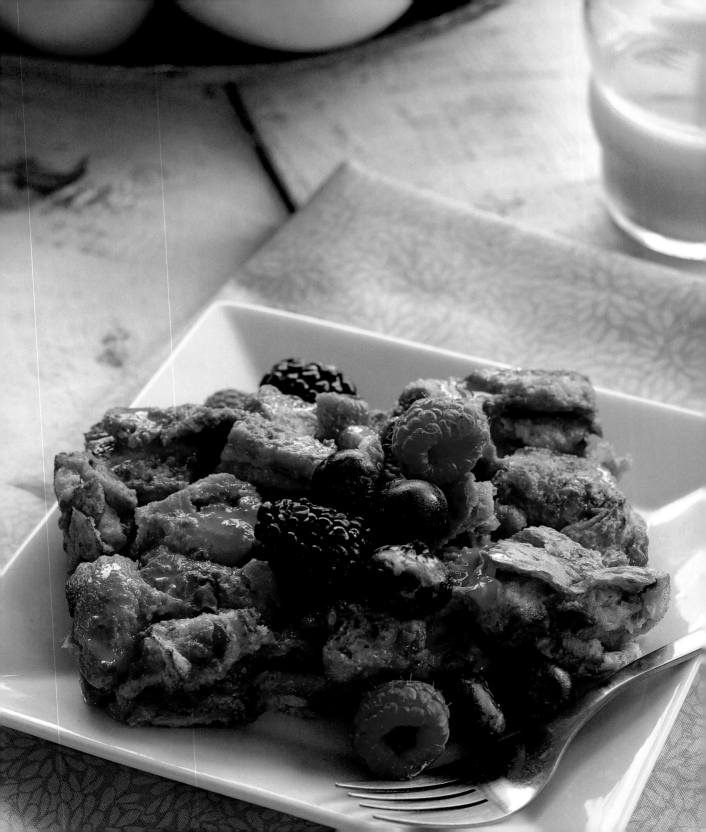

Cinnamon French Toast

Hope Comerford, Clinton Township, MI

Makes 8 servings
Prep. Time: 10 minutes ⚜ Cooking Time: 20 minutes ⚜ Setting: Manual
Pressure: High ⚜ Release: Natural then Manual

3 eggs

2 cups low-fat milk

2 tablespoons maple syrup

15 drops liquid stevia

2 teaspoons vanilla extract

2 teaspoons cinnamon

Pinch salt

16-ounces whole wheat bread, cubed and left out overnight to go stale

1½ cups water

Serving Suggestion:

Serve with a bit of fresh fruit on top, with an extra sprinkle of cinnamon.

1. In a medium bowl, whisk together the eggs, milk, maple syrup, Stevia, vanilla, cinnamon, and salt. Stir in the cubes of whole wheat bread.

2. You will need a 7-inch round baking pan for this. Spray the inside with nonstick spray, then pour the bread mixture into the pan.

3. Place the trivet in the bottom of the inner pot, then pour in the water.

4. Make foil sling and insert it onto the trivet. Carefully place the 7-inch pan on top of the foil sling/trivet.

5. Secure the lid to the locked position, then make sure the vent is turned to sealing.

6. Press the Manual button and use the "+/-" button to set the Instant Pot for 20 minutes.

7. When cook time is up, let the Instant Pot release naturally for 5 minutes, then quick release the rest.

Exchange List Values	Basic Nutritional Values	
Starch .5	Calories 75 (Calories from Fat 27)	Cholesterol 75 mg
Fat 0.5		Sodium 74 mg
	Total Fat 3 gm (Saturated Fat 1.3 gm, Polyunsat Fat 0.4 gm, Monounsat Fat 1.0 gm)	Total Carb 7 gm
		Dietary Fiber 0 gm
		Sugars 6 gm
		Protein 4.5 gm
		Phosphorus 99 mg

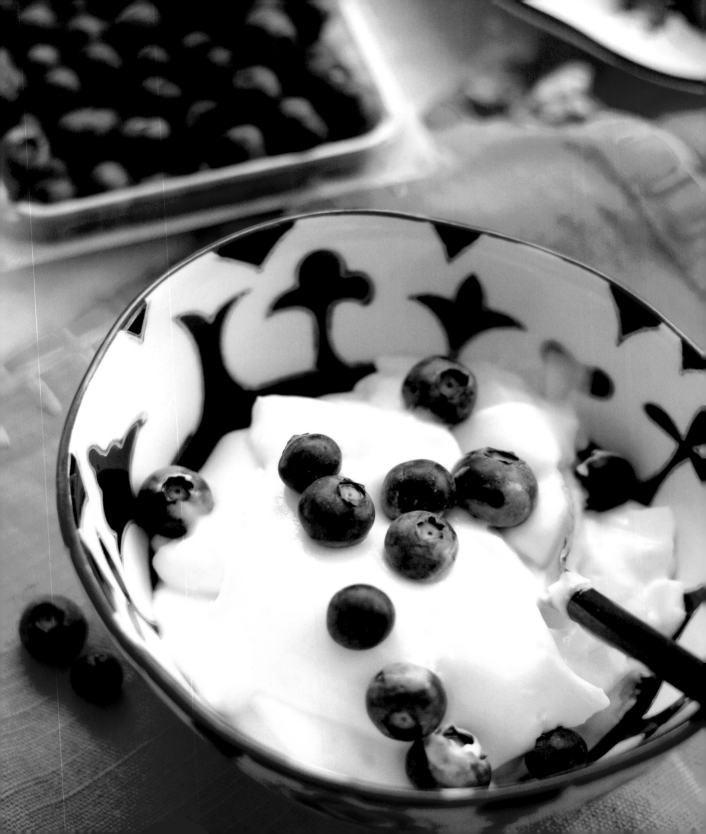

Cynthia's Yogurt

Cynthia Hockman-Chupp, Canby, OR

Makes 16 servings

Prep. Time: 10 minutes ⚜ Cooking Time: 8 hours+ ⚜ Setting: Yogurt

I gallon low-fat milk

¼ cup low-fat plain yogurt with active cultures

1. Pour milk into the inner pot of the Instant Pot.

2. Lock lid, move vent to sealing, and press the yogurt button. Press Adjust till it reads "boil."

3. When boil cycle is complete (about 1 hour), check the temperature. It should be at 185°F. If it's not, use the Sauté function to warm to 185.

4. After it reaches 185°F, unplug Instant Pot, remove inner pot, and cool. You can place on cooling rack and let it slowly cool. If in a hurry, submerge the base of the pot in cool water. Cool milk to 110°F.

5. When mixture reaches 110, stir in the ¼ cup of yogurt. Lock the lid in place and move vent to sealing.

6. Press Yogurt. Use the Adjust button until the screen says 8:00. This will now incubate for 8 hours.

7. After 8 hours (when the cycle is finished), chill yogurt, or go immediately to straining in step 8.

8. After chilling, or following the 8 hours, strain the yogurt using a nut milk bag. This will give it the consistency of Greek yogurt.

Serving suggestion:

When serving, top with fruit, granola, or nuts. If you'd like, add a dash of vanilla extract, peanut butter, or other flavoring. We also use this yogurt in smoothies!

Exchange List Values	Basic Nutritional Values	
Milk—low fat 1.0	Calories 141 (Calories from Fat 45)	Cholesterol 20 mg
Fat 1.0		Sodium 145 mg
	Total Fat 5 gm (Saturated Fat 3.0 gm, Polyunsat Fat 0.0 gm, Monounsat Fat 0.2 gm)	Total Carb 14 gm
		Dietary Fiber 0 gm
		Sugars 1 gm
		Protein 10 gm
		Phosphorus 279 mg

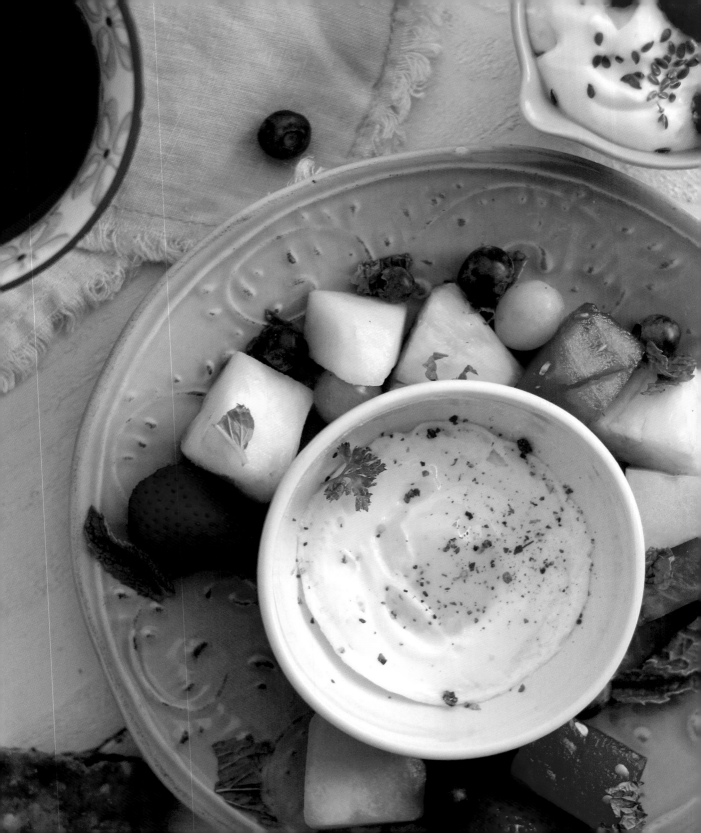

Poached Eggs

Hope Comerford, Clinton Township, MI

Makes 2–4 servings
Prep. Time: 5 minutes & Cooking Time: 2–5 minutes & Setting: Steam
Pressure: High & Release: Manual

1 cup water

4 large eggs

1. Place the trivet in the bottom of the inner pot of the Instant Pot and pour in the water.

2. You will need small silicone egg poacher cups that will fit in your Instant Pot to hold the eggs. Spray each silicone cup with nonstick cooking spray.

3. Crack each egg and pour it into the prepared cup.

4. Very carefully place the silicone cups into the Inner Pot so they do not spill.

5. Secure the lid by locking it into place and turn the vent to the sealing position.

6. Push the Steam button and adjust the time— 2 minutes for a very runny egg all the way to 5 minutes for a slightly runny egg.

7. When the timer beeps, release the pressure manually and remove the lid, being very careful not to let the condensation in the lid drip into your eggs.

8. Very carefully remove the silicone cups from the inner pot.

9. Carefully remove the poached eggs from each silicone cup and serve immediately.

Exchange List Values

Meat—medium fat 1.0

Basic Nutritional Values

Calories 72 (Calories from Fat 42)
Total Fat 5 gm (Saturated Fat 1.6 gm, Polyunsat Fat 1.0 gm, Monounsat Fat 1.8 gm)

Cholesterol 186 mg
Sodium 71 mg
Total Carb 0.4 gm
Dietary Fiber 0 gm
Sugars 0 gm
Protein 6 gm
Phosphorus 99 mg

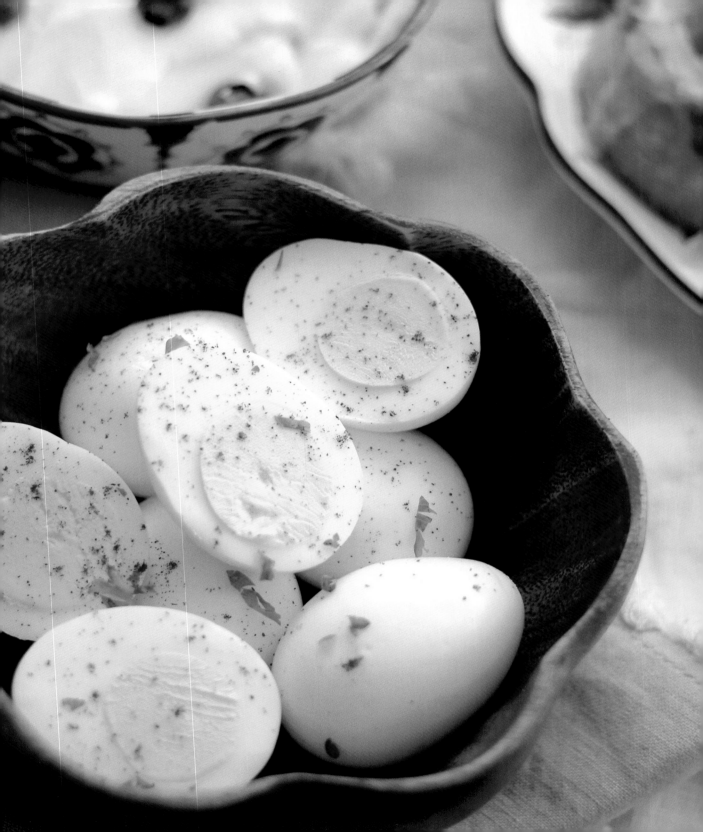

Instant Pot Hard-Boiled Eggs

Colleen Heatwole, Burton, MI

Makes 6–8 servings
Prep. Time: 10 minutes ☙ Cooking Time: 5 minutes ☙ Setting: Manual
Pressure: High ☙ Release: Manual

1 cup water
6–8 eggs

1. Pour the water into the inner pot. Place the eggs in a steamer basket or rack that came with pot.

2. Close the lid and secure to the locking position. Be sure the vent is turned to sealing. Set for 5 minutes on Manual at high pressure. (It takes about 5 minutes for pressure to build and then 5 minutes to cook.)

3. Let pressure naturally release for 5 minutes, then do quick pressure release.

4. Place hot eggs into cool water to halt cooking process. You can peel cooled eggs immediately or refrigerate unpeeled.

Exchange List Values

Meat—medium fat 1.0

Basic Nutritional Values

Calories 72 (Calories from Fat 42)
Total Fat 5 gm (Saturated Fat 1.6 gm, Polyunsat Fat 1.0 gm, Monounsat Fat 1.8 gm)

Cholesterol 186 mg
Sodium 71 mg
Total Carb 0.4 gm
Dietary Fiber 0 gm
Sugars 0 gm
Protein 6 gm
Phosphorus 99 mg

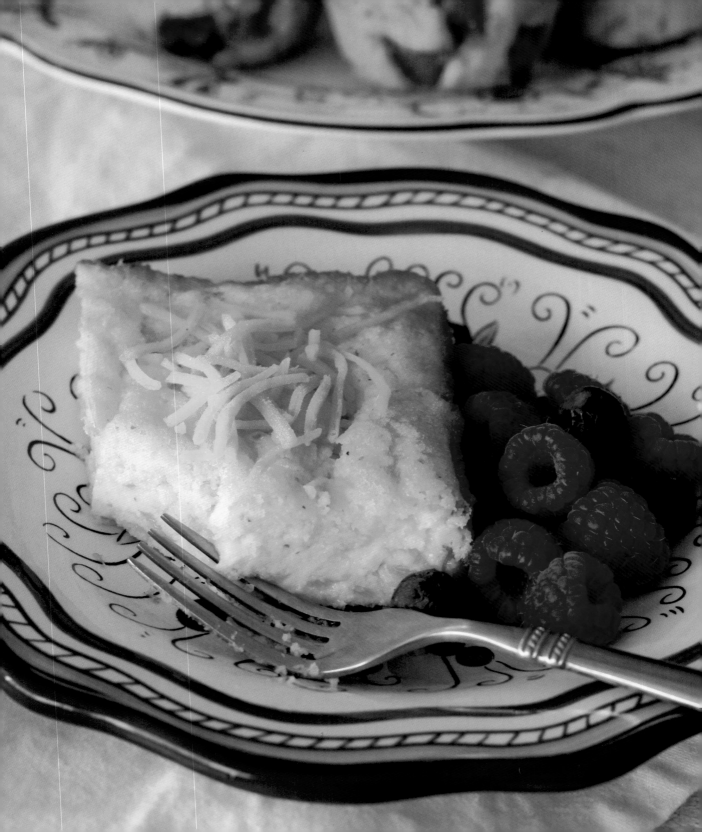

Baked Eggs

Esther J. Mast, Lancaster, PA

Make 8 servings
Prep. Time: 15 minutes ⚜ Cooking Time: 20 minutes ⚜ Setting: Manual
Pressure: High ⚜ Release: Natural

I cup water

2 tablespoons no-trans-fat tub margarine, melted

I cup reduced-fat buttermilk baking mix

1 ½ cups fat-free cottage cheese

2 teaspoons chopped onion

I teaspoon dried parsley

½ cup grated reduced-fat cheddar cheese

I egg, slightly beaten

1 ¼ cups egg substitute

I cup fat-free milk

Serving suggestion:

Serve with low-carb, low-sugar muffins and a fresh fruit cup.

1. Place the steaming rack into the bottom of the inner pot and pour in 1 cup of water.

2. Grease a round springform pan that will fit into the inner pot of the Instant Pot.

3. Pour melted margarine into springform pan.

4. Mix together buttermilk baking mix, cottage cheese, onion, parsley, cheese, egg, egg substitute, and milk in large mixing bowl.

5. Pour mixture over melted margarine. Stir slightly to distribute margarine.

6. Place the springform pan onto the steaming rack, close the lid, and secure to the locking position. Be sure the vent is turned to sealing. Set for 20 minutes on Manual at high pressure.

7. Let the pressure release naturally.

8. Carefully remove the springform pan with the handles of the steaming rack and allow to stand 10 minutes before cutting and serving.

Exchange List Values

Carbohydrate 1.0
Meat—lean 2.0

Basic Nutritional Values

Calories 155 (Calories from Fat 45)
Total Fat 5 gm
(Saturated Fat 1.5 gm, Trans Fat 0.0 gm, Polyunsat Fat 1.2 gm, Monounsat Fat 1.8 gm)

Cholesterol 30 mg
Sodium 460 mg
Potassium 195 gm
Total Carb 15 gm
Dietary Fiber 0 gm
Sugars 4 gm
Protein 12 gm
Phosphorus 250 gm

Easy Quiche

Becky Bontrager Horst, Goshen, IN

Makes 6 servings, 1 slice per serving
Prep. Time: 15 minutes ⚭ Cooking Time: 25 minutes ⚭ Setting: Manual
Pressure: High ⚭ Release: Natural

I cup water

¼ cup chopped onion

¼ cup chopped mushroom, *optional*

3 ounces 75%-less-fat cheddar cheese, shredded

2 tablespoons bacon bits, chopped ham or browned sausage

4 eggs

¼ teaspoons salt

I ½ cups fat-free milk

½ cup whole wheat flour

I tablespoon trans-fat-free tub margarine

1. Pour water into Instant Pot and place the steaming rack inside.

2. Spray a 6" round cake pan with nonstick spray.

3. Sprinkle the onion, mushroom, shredded cheddar, and meat around in the cake pan.

4. Combine remaining ingredients in medium bowl. Pour over meat and vegetables mixture.

5. Place the cake pan onto the steaming rack, close the lid and secure to the locking position. Be sure the vent is turned to sealing. Set for 25 minutes on Manual at high pressure.

7. Let the pressure release naturally.

8. Carefully remove the cake pan with the handles of the steaming rack and allow to stand 10 minutes before cutting and serving.

Exchange List Values

Meat—medium fat 1.5

Basic Nutritional Values

Calories 128 (Calories from Fat 45)
Total Fat 5 gm (Saturated Fat 1.5 gm, Polyunsat Fat 1.1 gm, Monounsat Fat 1.7 gm)

Cholesterol 127 mg
Sodium 302 mg
Total Carb 10 gm
Dietary Fiber 1 gm
Sugars 2 gm
Protein 11 gm
Phosphorus 209 mg

Potato-Bacon Gratin

Valerie Drobel, Carlisle, PA

Makes 8 servings, about 5 ounces per serving

Prep. Time: 20 minutes ⚜ Cooking Time: 40 minutes ⚜ Setting: Sauté and Manual
Pressure: High ⚜ Release: Quick

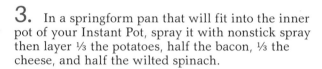

1 tablespoon olive oil

6-ounces bag fresh spinach

1 clove garlic, minced

4 large potatoes, peeled or unpeeled, *divided*

6-ounces Canadian bacon slices, *divided*

5-ounces reduced-fat grated Swiss cheddar, *divided*

1 cup lower-sodium, lower-fat chicken broth

1. Set the Instant Pot to Sauté and pour in the olive oil. Cook the spinach and garlic in olive oil just until spinach is wilted (5 minutes or less). Turn off the instant pot.

2. Cut potatoes into thin slices about ¼" thick.

3. In a springform pan that will fit into the inner pot of your Instant Pot, spray it with nonstick spray then layer ⅓ the potatoes, half the bacon, ⅓ the cheese, and half the wilted spinach.

4. Repeat layers ending with potatoes. Reserve ⅓ cheese for later.

5. Pour chicken broth over all.

6. Wipe the bottom of your Instant Pot to soak up any remaining oil, then add in 2 cups of water and the steaming rack. Place the springform pan on top.

7. Close the lid and secure to the locking position. Be sure the vent is turned to sealing. Set for 35 minutes on Manual at high pressure.

8. Perform a quick release.

9. Top with the remaining cheese, then allow to stand 10 minutes before removing from the Instant Pot, cutting and serving.

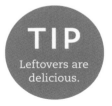

TIP
Leftovers are delicious.

Exchange List Values

Carbohydrate 2.0
Meat—lean 2.0

Basic Nutritional Values

Calories 220 (Calories from Fat 65)
Total Fat 7 gm (Saturated Fat 2.4 gm, Trans Fat 0.0 gm, Polyunsat Fat 0.5 gm, Monounsat Fat 2.7 gm)

Cholesterol 25 mg
Sodium 415 mg
Potassium 710 gm
Total Carb 28 gm
Dietary Fiber 3 gm
Sugars 2 gm
Protein 14 gm
Phosphorus 285 gm

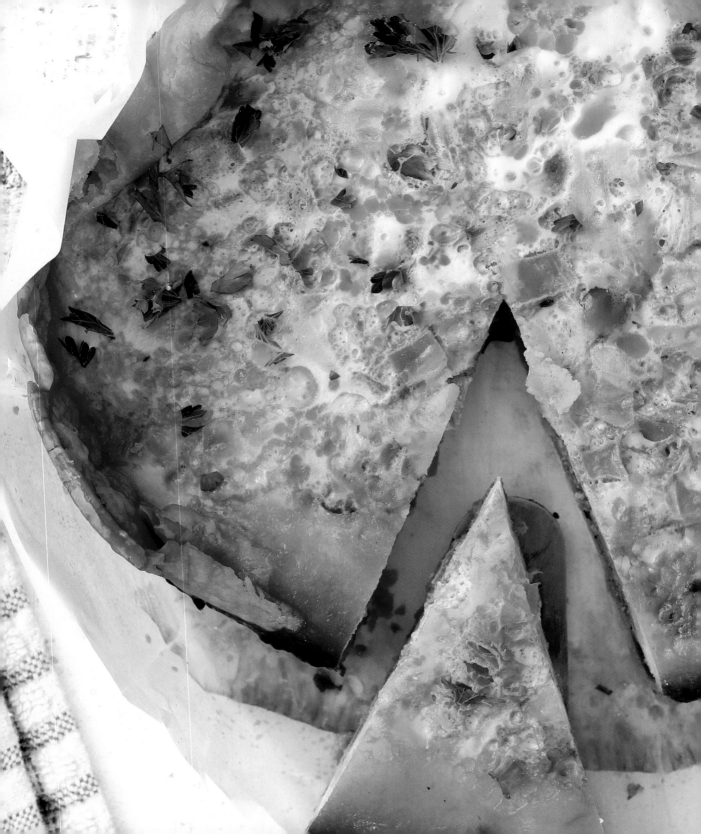

Southwestern Egg Casserole

Eileen Eash, Lafayette, CO

Makes 12 servings

Prep. Time: 10 minutes ⚬ Cooking Time: 20 minutes ⚬ Setting: Manual
Pressure: High ⚬ Release: Natural

1 cup water

2½ cups egg substitute

½ cup flour

1 teaspoon baking powder

⅛ teaspoon salt

⅛ teaspoon pepper

2 cups fat-free cottage cheese

1½ cups shredded 75%-less-fat sharp cheddar cheese

¼ cup no-trans-fat tub margarine, melted

2 (4-ounce) cans chopped green chilies

1. Place the steaming rack into the bottom of the inner pot and pour in 1 cup of water.

2. Grease a round springform pan that will fit into the inner pot of the Instant Pot.

3. Combine the egg substitute, flour, baking powder, salt and pepper in a mixing bowl. It will be lumpy.

4. Stir in the cheese, margarine, and green chilies then pour into the springform pan.

5. Place the springform pan onto the steaming rack, close the lid, and secure to the locking position. Be sure the vent is turned to sealing. Set for 20 minutes on Manual at high pressure.

6. Let the pressure release naturally.

7. Carefully remove the springform pan with the handles of the steaming rack and allow to stand 10 minutes before cutting and serving.

Exchange List Values

Carbohydrate 0.5
Meat—lean 2.0

Basic Nutritional Values

Calories 130 (Calories from Fat 35)
Total Fat 4 gm (Saturated Fat 1.4 gm, Trans Fat 0.0 gm, Polyunsat Fat 1.2 gm, Monounsat Fat 1.2 gm)

Cholesterol 10 mg
Sodium 450 mg
Potassium 180 gm
Total Carb 9 gm
Dietary Fiber 1 gm
Sugars 1 gm
Protein 14 gm
Phosphorus 190 gm

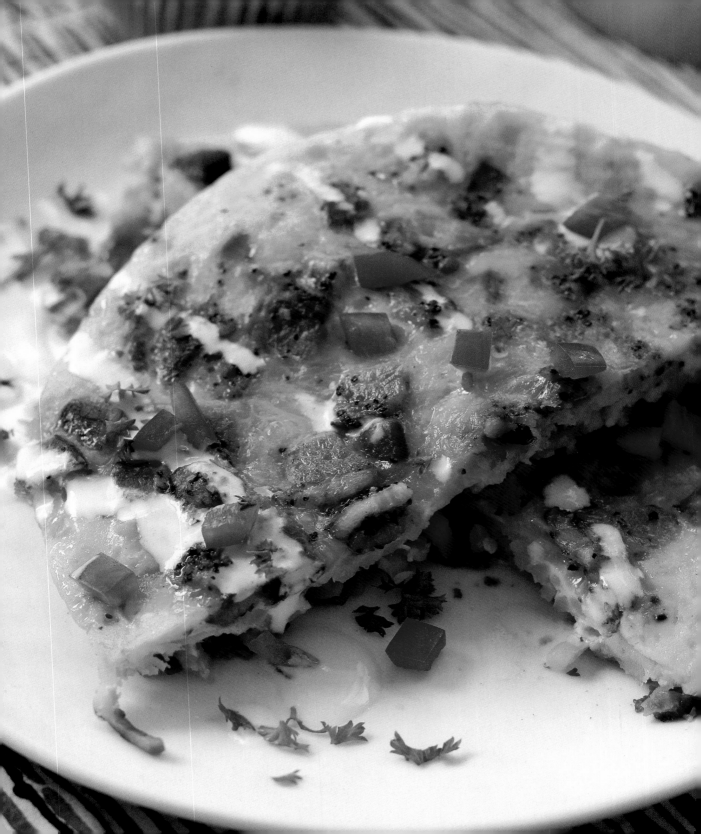

Shredded Potato Omelet

Mary H. Nolt, East Earl, PA

Makes 6 servings

Prep. Time: 15 minutes ⚭ Cooking Time: 20 minutes ⚭ Setting: Manual
Pressure: High ⚭ Release: Natural

3 slices bacon, cooked and crumbled

2 cups shredded cooked potatoes

¼ cup minced onion

¼ cup minced green bell pepper

1 cup egg substitute

¼ cup fat-free milk

¼ teaspoon salt

⅛ teaspoon black pepper

1 cup 75%-less-fat shredded cheddar cheese

1 cup water

1. With nonstick cooking spray, spray the inside of a round baking dish that will fit in your Instant Pot inner pot.

2. Sprinkle the bacon, potatoes, onion, and bell pepper around the bottom of the baking dish.

3. Mix together the egg substitute, milk, salt, and pepper in mixing bowl. Pour over potato mixture.

4. Top with cheese.

5. Add water, place the steaming rack into the bottom of the inner pot and then place the round baking dish on top.

6. Close the lid and secure to the locking position. Be sure the vent is turned to sealing. Set for 20 minutes on Manual at high pressure.

7. Let the pressure release naturally.

8. Carefully remove the baking dish with the handles of the steaming rack and allow to stand 10 minutes before cutting and serving.

Exchange List Values

Starch 1.0

Meat—lean 1.0

Basic Nutritional Values

Calories 130 (Calories from Fat 25)

Total Fat 3 gm (Saturated Fat 1.4 gm, Trans Fat 0.0 gm, Polyunsat Fat 0.2 gm, Monounsat Fat 0.9 gm)

Cholesterol 10 mg

Sodium 415 mg

Potassium 280 gm

Total Carb 13 gm

Dietary Fiber 2 gm

Sugars 2 gm

Protein 12 gm

Phosphorus 150 gm

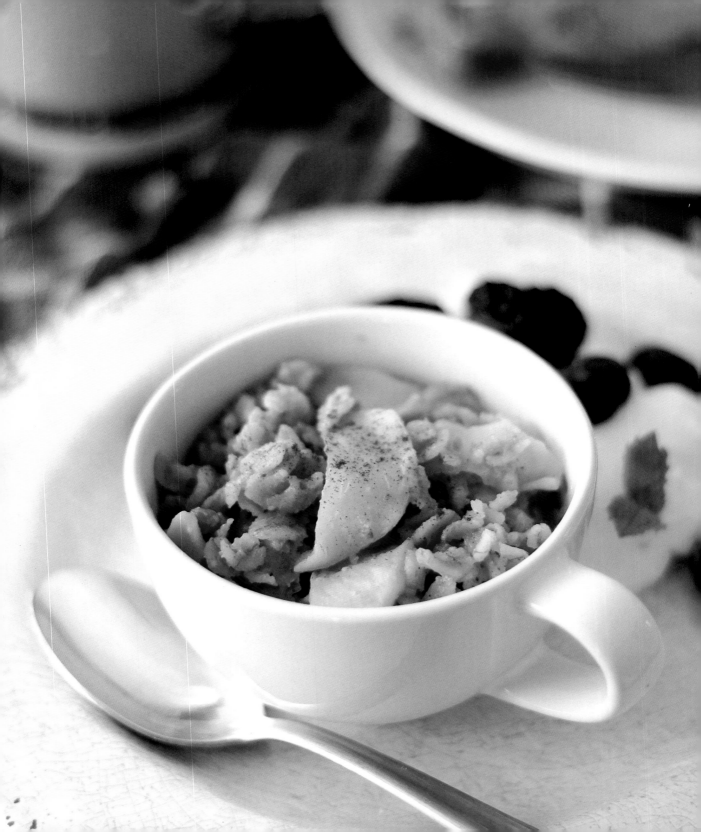

Apple Oatmeal

Frances B. Musser
Newmanstown, PA

Makes 6 servings
Prep. Time: 20 minutes ⚜ *Cooking Time: 8 minutes* ⚜ *Setting: Manual*
Pressure: High ⚜ *Release: Natural then Manual*

2 cups water
2 cups fat-free milk
1½ tablespoons honey
1 tablespoon light, soft tub margarine
¼ teaspoon salt
1 teaspoon cinnamon
2 cups dry rolled oats
1 cup chopped apples
½ cup chopped walnuts
1 tablespoon brown sugar
brown sugar substitute to equal ½ tablespoons sugar

1. Place the steaming rack into the inner pot of the Instant pot and pour in the 1 cup of water.

2. In an approximately 7-cup heat-safe baking dish, add all of your ingredients, including remaining 1 cup of water, and stir.

3. Place the dish on top of the steaming rack, close the lid, and secure it to a locking position.

4. Be sure the vent is set to sealing, then set the Instant Pot for 8 minutes on Manual.

5. When it is done cooking, allow the pressure to release naturally for 5 minutes and then perform a quick release.

6. Carefully remove the rack and dish from the Instant Pot and serve.

Exchange List Values

Starch 1.5
Fat 2.0
Fruit 1.0

Basic Nutritional Values

Calories 267 (Calories from Fat 99)
Total Fat 11 gm (Saturated Fat 1.3 gm, Polyunsat Fat 5.1 gm, Monounsat Fat 1.8 gm)

Cholesterol 2 mg
Sodium 140 mg
Total Carb 36 gm
Dietary Fiber 0 gm
Sugars 5 gm
Protein 13 gm
Phosphorus 120 mg

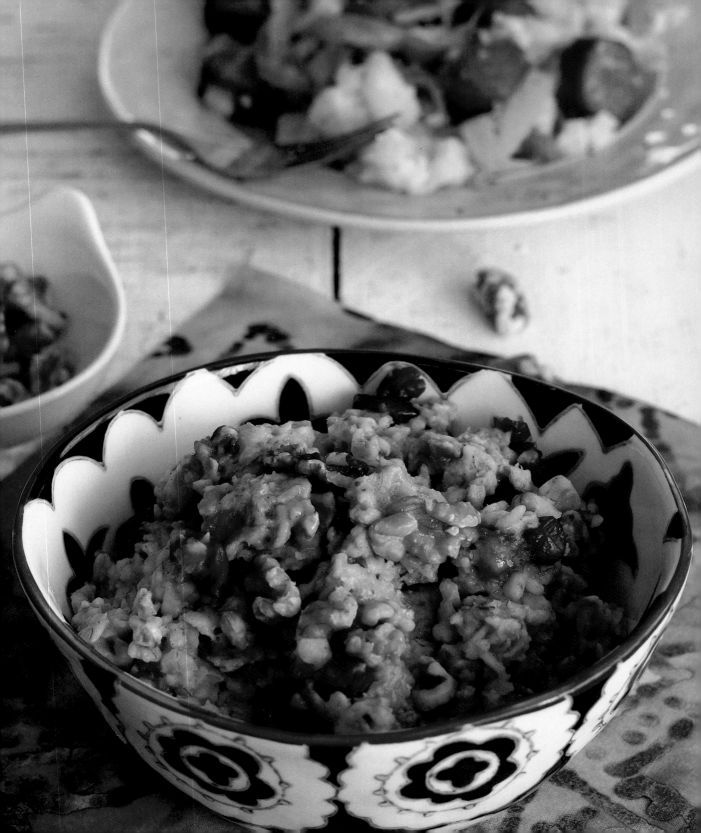

Oatmeal Morning

Barbara Forrester Landis, Lititz, PA

Makes 6 servings
Prep. Time: 5 minutes ⚜ Cooking Time: 4 minutes ⚜ Setting: Manual
Pressure: High ⚜ Release: Natural

I cup water
2 cups uncooked steel cut oats
I cup dried cranberries
I cup walnuts
½ teaspoon salt
I tablespoon cinnamon
I cup water
2 cups fat-free milk

1. Place the steaming rack into the inner pot of the Instant pot and pour in the 1 cup of water.

2. In an approximately 7-cup heat-safe baking dish, add all of your ingredients and stir.

3. Place the dish on top of the steaming rack, close the lid, and secure it to a locking position.

4. Be sure the vent is set to sealing, then set the Instant Pot for 4 minutes on Manual.

5. When it is done cooking, allow the pressure to release naturally.

6. Carefully remove the rack and dish from the Instant Pot and serve.

Exchange List Values

Starch 4.0
Fat 2.0

Basic Nutritional Values

Calories 383 (Calories from Fat 90)
Total Fat 10 gm (Saturated Fat 1.3 gm, Polyunsat Fat 4.6 gm, Monounsat Fat 1.0 gm)

Cholesterol 2 mg
Sodium 197 mg
Total Carb 62 gm
Dietary Fiber 9 gm
Sugars 19 gm
Protein 14 gm
Phosphorus 119 mg

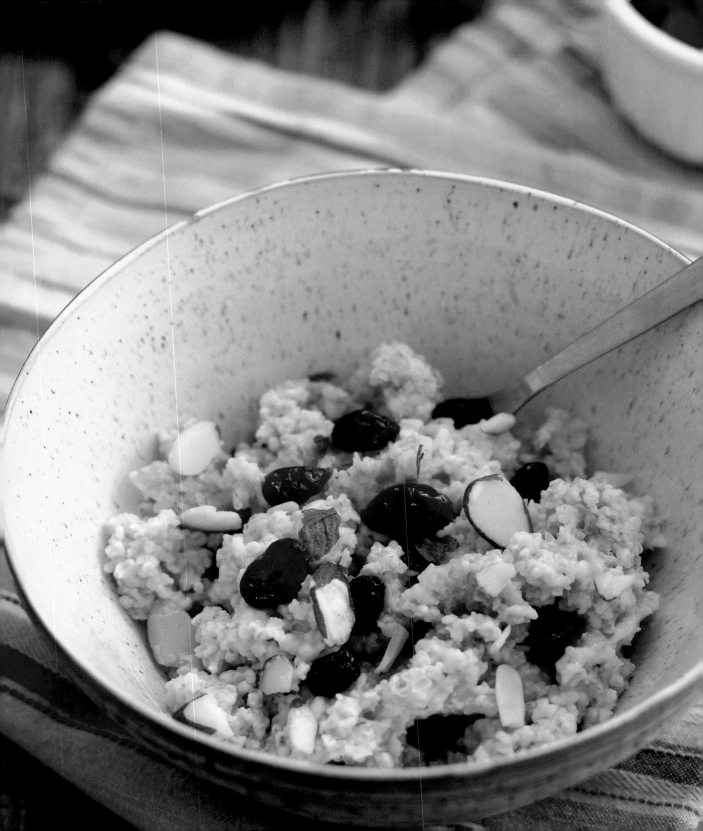

Best Steel-Cut Oats

Colleen Heatwole, Burton, MI

Makes 4 servings
Prep. Time: 5 minutes ⚜ Cooking Time: 3 minutes ⚜ Setting: Manual
Pressure: High ⚜ Release: Natural

I cup steel-cut oats

2 cups water

I cup unsweetened almond milk

Pinch salt

½ teaspoons vanilla extract

I cinnamon stick

¼ cup raisins

¼ cup dried cherries

I teaspoon ground cinnamon

¼ cup toasted almonds

Sweetener of choice, *optional*

1. Add all ingredients to the inner pot of the Instant Pot except the toasted almonds and sweetener.

2. Secure the lid and make sure the vent is turned to sealing. Cook 3 minutes on high, using Manual function.

3. Let the pressure release naturally.

4. Remove cinnamon stick.

5. Add almonds, and sweetener if desired, and serve.

NOTE

Refrigerate leftovers in refrigerator.

Nondairy milk is best because dairy milk can scorch. Additional milk can be added when eating if desired.

This is supposed to serve 4 but rarely serves more than 2 at our house.

We never add additional sweetener.

Exchange List Values

Starch 3.0

Fat 1.5

Basic Nutritional Values

Calories 276 (Calories from Fat 60)

Total Fat 7 gm (Saturated Fat 0.7 gm, Polyunsat Fat 0.8 gm, Monounsat Fat 2.3 gm)

Cholesterol 0 mg

Sodium 53 mg

Total Carb 46 gm

Dietary Fiber 7 gm

Sugars 12 gm

Protein 9 gm

Phosphorus 47 mg

Appetizers & Snacks

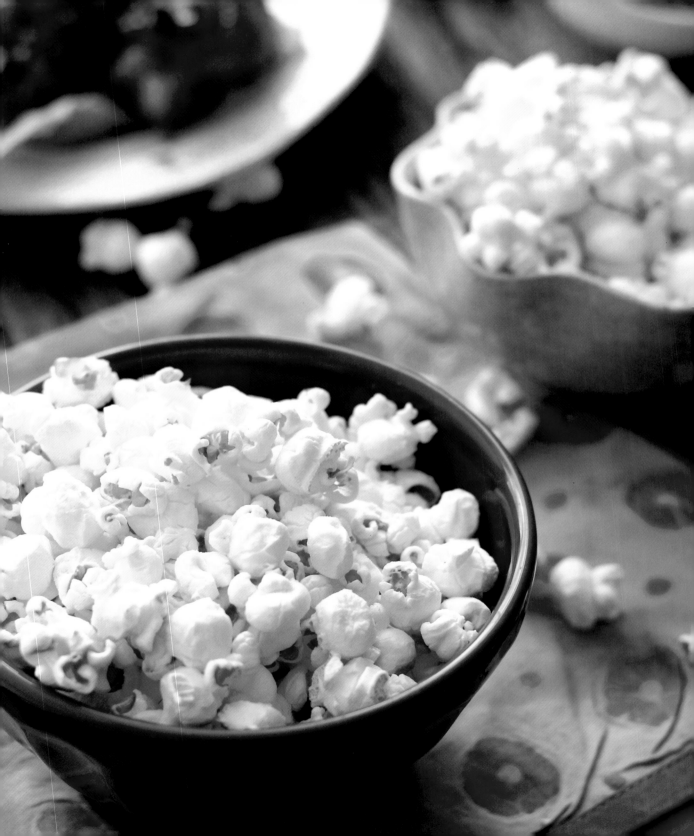

Insta Popcorn

Hope Comerford, Clinton Township, MI

Makes 5–6 servings
Prep. Time: 1 minute & Cooking Time: about 5 minutes & Setting: Sauté

2 tablespoons coconut oil

½ cup popcorn kernels

¼ cup margarine spread, melted, *optional*

Sea salt to taste

1. Set the Instant Pot to Sauté.

2. Melt the coconut oil in the inner pot, then add the popcorn kernels and stir.

3. Press Adjust to bring the temperature up to high.

4. When the corn starts popping, secure the lid on the Instant Pot.

5. When you no longer hear popping, turn off the Instant Pot, remove the lid, and pour the popcorn into a bowl.

6. Top with the optional melted margarine and season the popcorn with sea salt to your liking.

Exchange List Values

Starch 1.0

Fat 2.5

Basic Nutritional Values

Calories 161 (Calories from Fat 108)

Total Fat 12 gm (Saturated Fat 5.2 gm, Polyunsat Fat 2.8 gm, Monounsat Fat 3.9 gm)

Cholesterol 0 mg

Sodium 89 mg

Potassium 2.8 gm

Total Carb 13 gm

Dietary Fiber 3 gm

Sugars 0 gm

Protein 1 gm

Phosphorus 2 mg

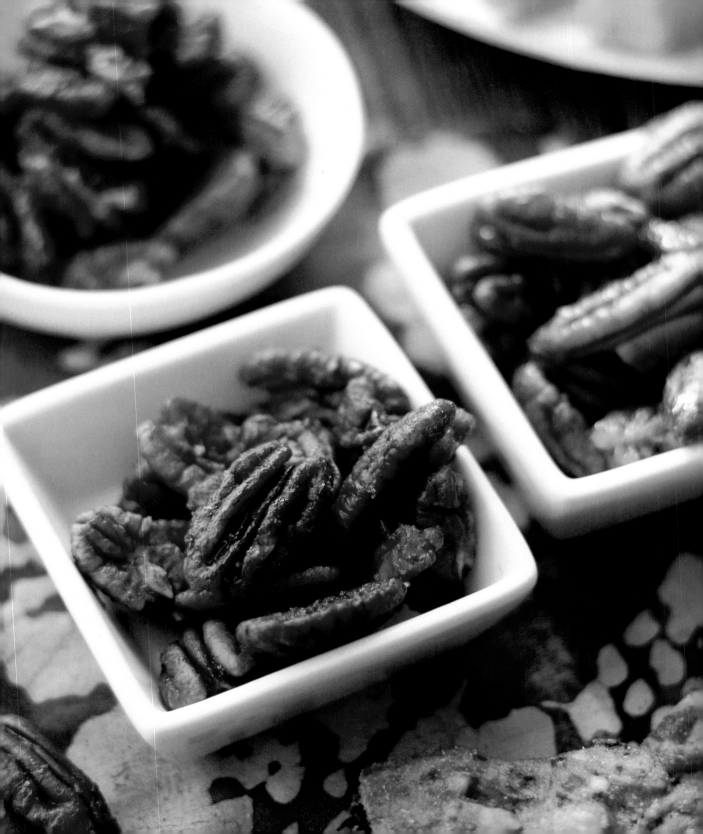

Candied Pecans

Hope Comerford, Clinton Township, MI

Makes 10 servings

Prep. Time: 5 minutes ⚬ Cooking Time: 20 minutes ⚬ Setting: Sauté and Manual
Pressure: High ⚬ Release: Manual

4 cups raw pecans
1 ½ teaspoons liquid stevia
½ cup plus 1 tablespoon water, *divided*
1 teaspoon vanilla extract
1 teaspoon cinnamon
¼ teaspoon nutmeg
⅛ teaspoon ground ginger
⅛ teaspoon sea salt

1. Place the raw pecans, liquid stevia, 1 tablespoon water, vanilla, cinnamon, nutmeg, ground ginger, and sea salt into the inner pot of the Instant Pot.

2. Press the Sauté button on the Instant Pot and sauté the pecans and other ingredients until the pecans are soft.

3. Pour in the ½ cup water and secure the lid to the locked position. Set the vent to sealing.

4. Press Manual and set the Instant Pot for 15 minutes.

5. Preheat the oven to 350°F.

6. When cooking time is up, turn off the Instant Pot, then do a quick release.

7. Spread the pecans onto a greased, lined baking sheet.

8. Bake the pecans for 5 minutes or less in the oven, checking on them frequently so they do not burn.

NOTE

These can be kept at room temperature in a tightly sealed container (after completely cooled) for about a week. You could also store these in the refrigerator in a tightly sealed container for about 4 weeks.

Exchange List Values

Fat 6.0

Basic Nutritional Values

Calories 275 (Calories from Fat 256)
Total Fat 28.5 gm
(Saturated Fat 2.5 gm, Polyunsat Fat 86 gm, Monounsat Fat 16.2 gm)

Cholesterol 0 mg
Sodium 20 mg
Potassium 164 mg
Total Carb 6 gm
Dietary Fiber 4 gm
Sugars 2 gm
Protein 4 gm
Phosphorus 110 mg

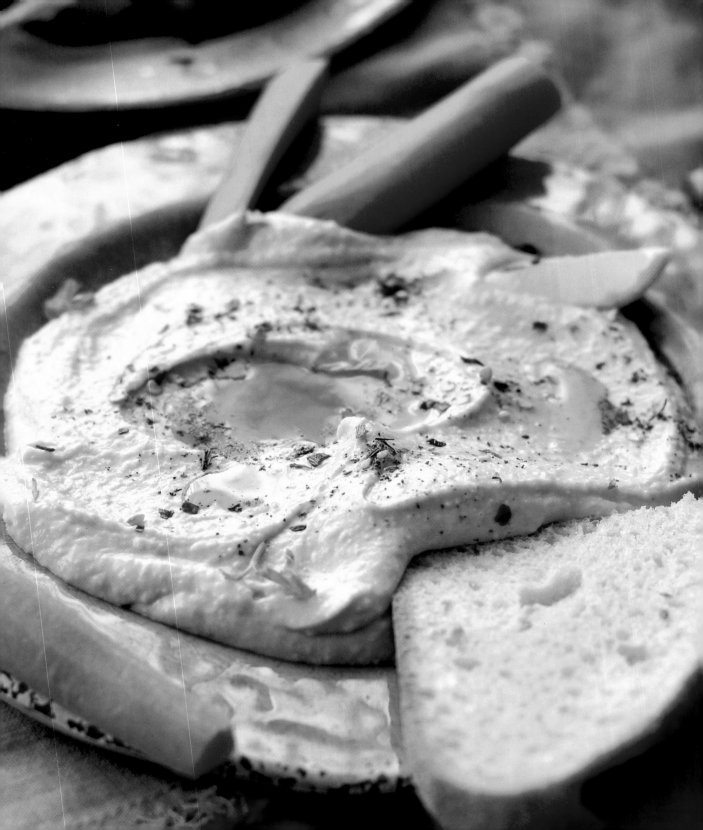

Hummus

Colleen Heatwole, Burton, MI

Makes 8 servings
Prep. Time: 15 minutes & Cooking Time: 40 minutes & Setting: Manual or Bean
Pressure: High & Release: Natural

1 cup dry garbanzo beans (chickpeas)
4 cups water
2 tablespoons fresh lemon juice
¼ cup chopped onion
3 cloves garlic, minced
½ cup tahini (sesame paste)
2 teaspoons olive oil
2 teaspoons cumin
Pinch cayenne pepper
½ teaspoon salt, *optional*

Serving suggestion:
Serve with vegetable crudités, whole wheat pita, or whole grain crackers.

1. Place garbanzo beans and 4 cups water into inner pot of Instant Pot. Secure lid and make sure vent is set to sealing.

2. Cook garbanzo beans and water for 40 minutes using the Manual high pressure setting.

3. When cooking time is up, let the pressure release naturally.

4. Test the garbanzos. If still firm, cook using Slow Cook function until they are soft.

5. Drain the garbanzo beans, but save ½ cup of the cooking liquid.

6. Combine the garbanzos, lemon juice, onion, garlic, tahini, oil, cumin, pepper, and optional salt in a blender or food processor.

7. Puree until smooth, adding chickpea liquid as needed to thin the puree. Taste and adjust seasonings accordingly.

Exchange List Values
Meat 0.5
Fat 1.0

Basic Nutritional Values
Calories 200 (Calories from Fat 99)
Total Fat 11 gm (Saturated Fat 1.4 gm, Polyunsat Fat 4.2 gm, Monounsat Fat 4.2 gm)

Cholesterol 0 mg
Sodium 16 mg
Potassium 276 gm
Total Carb 20 gm
Dietary Fiber 4 gm
Sugars 3 gm
Protein 8 gm
Phosphorus 185 mg

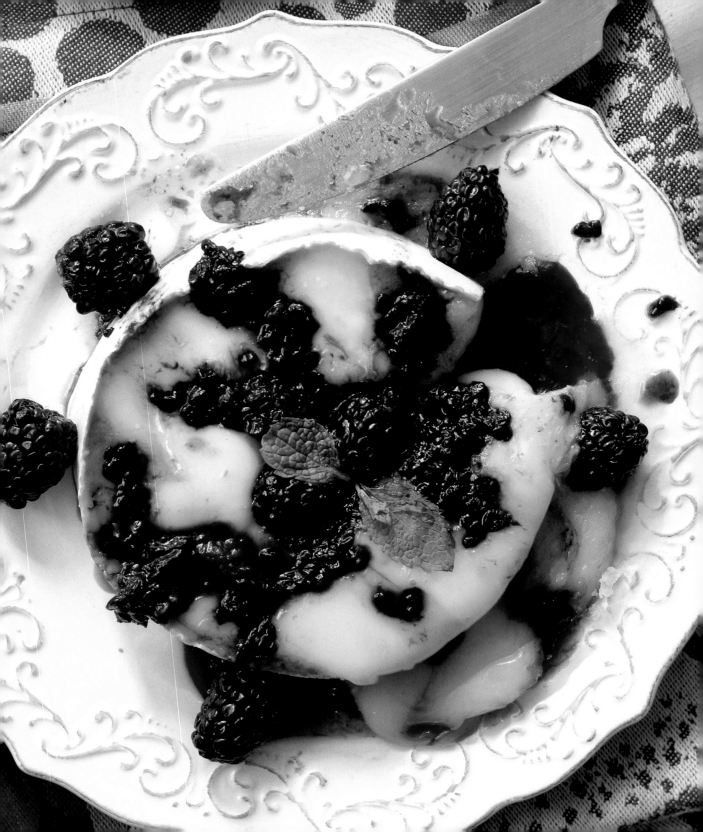

Blackberry Baked Brie

Hope Comerford, Clinton Township, MI

Makes 4–6 servings
Prep. Time: 5 minutes ⚜ Cooking Time: 15 minutes ⚜ Setting: Manual
Pressure: High ⚜ Release: Manual

8-ounce round Brie

1 cup water

¼ cup sugar-free blackberry preserves

2 teaspoons chopped fresh mint

1. Slice a grid pattern into the top of the rind of the Brie with a knife.

2. In a 7-inch round baking dish, place the Brie, then cover the baking dish securely with foil.

3. Insert the trivet into the inner pot of the Instant Pot; pour in the water.

4. Make a foil sling and arrange it on top of the trivet. Place the baking dish on top of the trivet and foil sling.

5. Secure the lid to the locked position and turn the vent to sealing.

6. Press Manual and set the Instant Pot for 15 minutes on high pressure.

7. When cooking time is up, turn off the Instant Pot and do a quick release of the pressure.

8. When the valve has dropped, remove the lid, then remove the baking dish.

9. Remove the top rind of the Brie and top with the preserves. Sprinkle with the fresh mint.

Serving suggestion:
Serve with whole grain crostini or whole grain crackers.

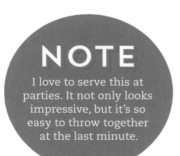

NOTE

I love to serve this at parties. It not only looks impressive, but it's so easy to throw together at the last minute.

Exchange List Values

Fat 2.0

Basic Nutritional Values

Calories 133 (Calories from Fat 90)
Total Fat 10 gm (Saturated Fat 6.7 gm, Polyunsat Fat 0.3 gm, Monounsat Fat 3.0 gm)
Cholesterol 38 mg
Sodium 238 mg
Potassium 59 gm
Total Carb 4 gm
Dietary Fiber 0 gm
Sugars 0 gm
Protein 8 gm
Phosphorus 71 mg

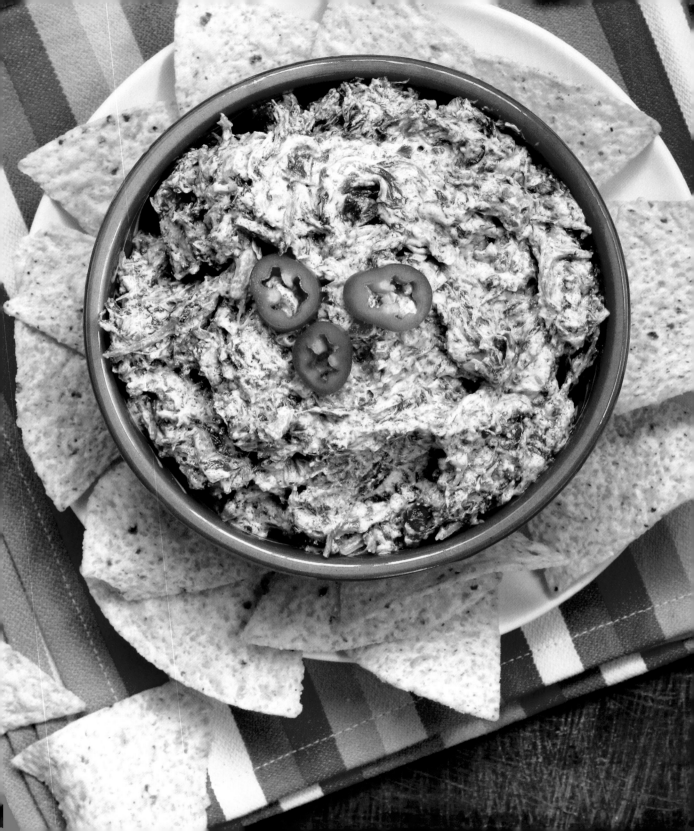

Creamy Spinach Dip

Jessica Stoner, Arlington, OH

Makes 10–12 servings
Prep. Time: 10–15 minutes ⚜ Cooking Time: 5 minutes ⚜ Setting: Bean/Chili
Pressure: High ⚜ Release: Manual

8 ounces low-fat cream cheese
1 cup low-fat sour cream
½ cup finely chopped onion
½ cup no-sodium vegetable broth
5 cloves garlic, minced
½ teaspoon salt
¼ teaspoon black pepper
10 ounces frozen spinach
12 ounces reduced-fat shredded Monterey Jack cheese
12 ounces reduced-fat shredded Parmesan cheese

1. Add cream cheese, sour cream, onion, vegetable broth, garlic, salt, pepper, and spinach to the inner pot of the Instant Pot.

2. Secure lid, make sure vent is set to sealing, and set to the Bean/Chili setting on high pressure for 5 minutes.

3. When done, do a manual release.

4. Add the cheeses and mix well until creamy and well combined.

Serving suggestion:
Serve with whole grain tortilla chips or whole grain bread.

Exchange List Values

Milk—whole 1.0
Fat 3.5

Basic Nutritional Values

Calories 274 (Calories from Fat 162)
Total Fat 18 gm (Saturated Fat 10.4 gm, Polyunsat Fat 0.8 gm, Monounsat Fat 4.3 gm)

Cholesterol 56 mg
Sodium 948 mg
Potassium 219 gm
Total Carb 10 gm
Dietary Fiber 1 gm
Sugars 3 gm
Protein 19 gm
Phosphorus 219 mg

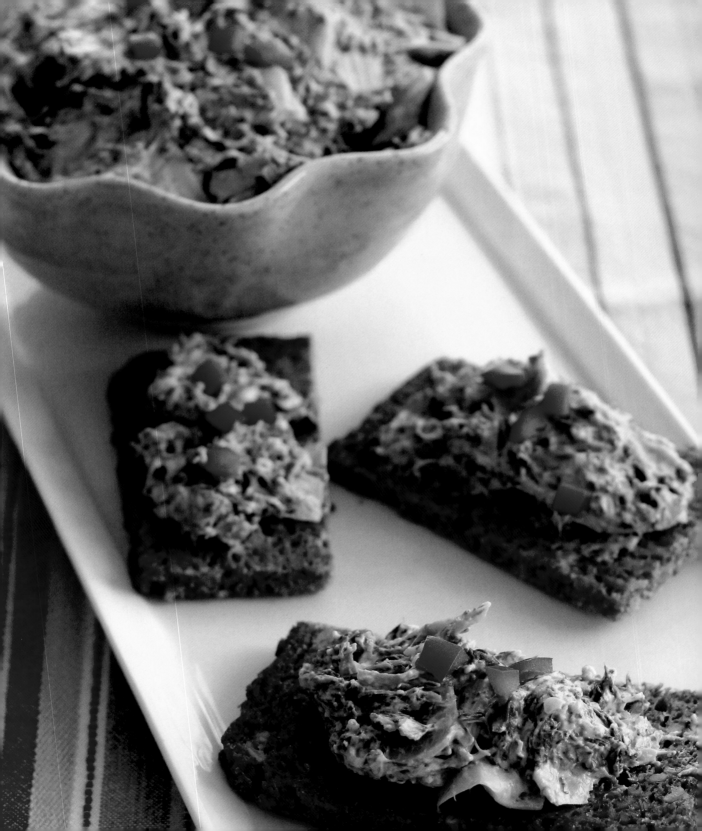

Spinach and Artichoke Dip

Michele Ruvola, Vestal, NY

Makes 10–12 servings
Prep. Time: 5 minutes & Cooking Time: 4 minutes & Setting: Manual
Pressure: High & Release: Manual

8 ounces low-fat cream cheese
10-ounce box frozen spinach
½ cup no-sodium chicken broth
14-ounce can artichoke hearts, drained
½ cup low-fat sour cream
½ cup low-fat mayo
3 cloves of garlic, minced
1 teaspoon onion powder
16 ounces reduced-fat shredded Parmesan cheese
8 ounces reduced-fat shredded mozzarella

1. Put all ingredients in the inner pot of the Instant Pot, except the Parmesan cheese and the mozzarella cheese.

2. Secure the lid and set vent to sealing. Place on Manual high pressure for 4 minutes.

3. Do a quick release of steam.

4. Immediately stir in the cheeses.

Serving suggestion:

Serve with vegetables or sliced whole grain bread.

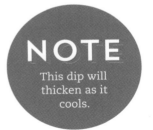

NOTE
This dip will thicken as it cools.

Exchange List Values

Milk—whole 1.0
Fat 3.5

Basic Nutritional Values

Calories 288 (Calories from Fat 162)
Total Fat 18 gm
(Saturated Fat 9.7 gm, Polyunsat Fat 0.7 gm, Monounsat Fat 3.5 gm)

Cholesterol 54 mg
Sodium 1007 mg
Potassium 300 gm
Total Carb 15 gm
Dietary Fiber 3 gm
Sugars 3 gm
Protein 19 gm
Phosphorus 303 mg

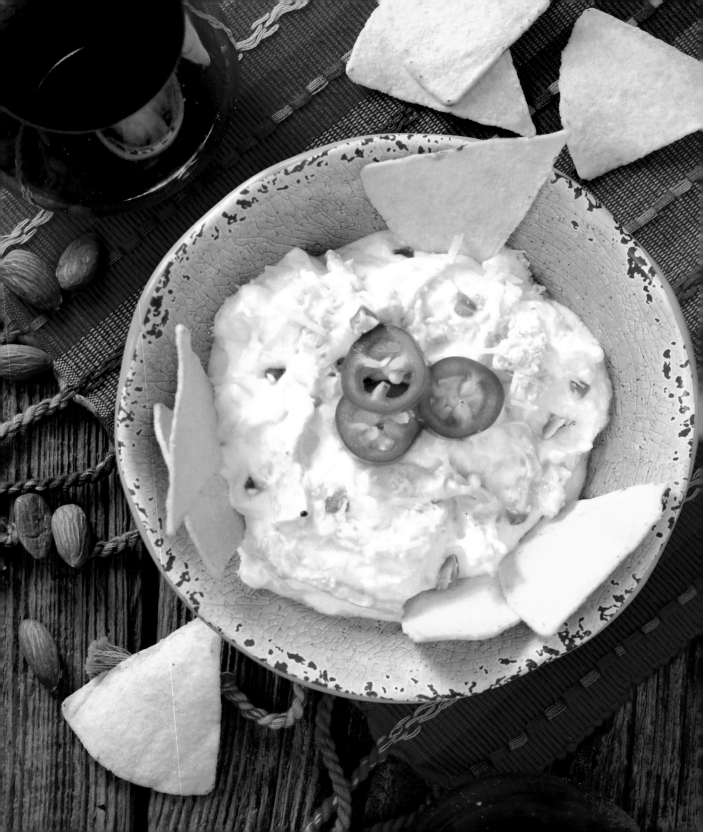

Creamy Jalapeño Chicken Dip

Hope Comerford, Clinton Township, MI

Makes 10 servings

Prep. Time: 5 minutes   ☙   Cooking Time: 12 minutes   ☙   Setting: Manual
Pressure: High   ☙   Release: Manual

1 pound boneless chicken breast

8 ounces low-fat cream cheese

3 jalapeños, seeded and sliced

½ cup water

8 ounces reduced-fat shredded cheddar cheese

¾ cup low-fat sour cream

1. Place the chicken, cream cheese, jalapeños, and water in the inner pot of the Instant Pot.

2. Secure the lid so it's locked and turn the vent to sealing.

3. Press Manual and set the Instant Pot for 12 minutes on high pressure.

4. When cooking time is up, turn off Instant Pot, do a quick release of the remaining pressure, then remove lid.

5. Shred the chicken between 2 forks, either in the pot or on a cutting board, then place back in the inner pot.

6. Stir in the shredded cheese and sour cream.

Exchange List Values

Meat—medium fat 3.5

Basic Nutritional Values

Calories 238 (Calories from Fat 117)
Total Fat 13 gm (Saturated Fat 6.8 gm, Polyunsat Fat 0.7 gm, Monounsat Fat 1.7 gm)

Cholesterol 75 mg
Sodium 273 mg
Potassium 310 mg
Total Carb 7 gm
Dietary Fiber 1 gm
Sugars 5 gm
Protein 24 gm
Phosphorus 159 mg

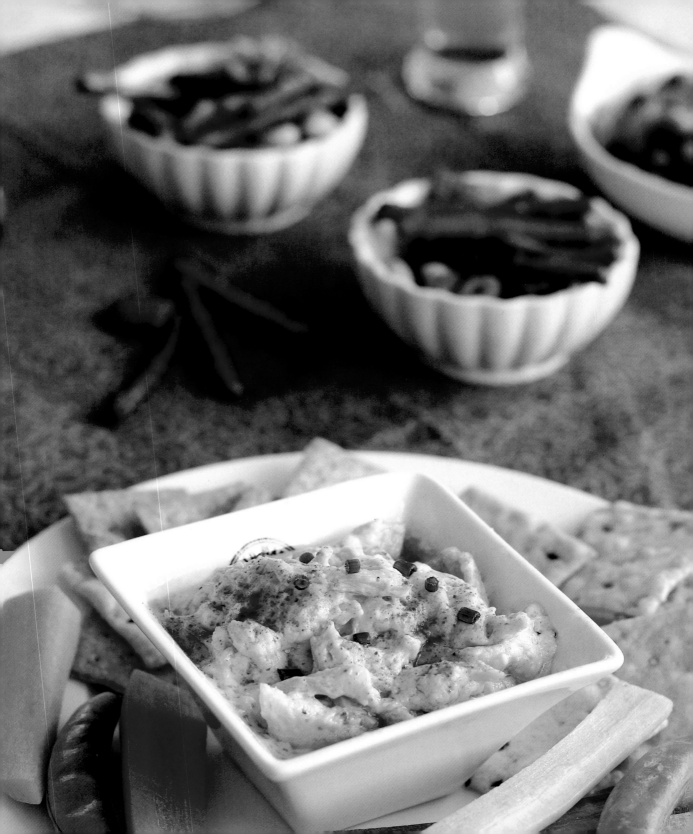

Buffalo Chicken Dip

Hope Comerford, Clinton Township, MI

Makes 26 servings
Prep. Time: 15 minutes & Cook Time: 15 minutes & Setting: Manual then Sauté
Pressure: High & Release: Natural then Manual

2 large frozen boneless skinless chicken breasts

¾ cup Frank's RedHot sauce

½ cup sodium-free chicken broth

1 cup light ranch dressing

2 (8-ounce) packages fat-free cream cheese, softened

1 ½ cups reduced-fat shredded cheddar jack cheese

1. Place the frozen chicken, hot sauce, and chicken broth into the inner pot of the Instant Pot. Secure the lid and make sure the vent is set to sealing.

2. Set the Instant Pot for 10 minutes on Manual. When cooking time is over, let the pressure release naturally for 10 minutes and then perform a quick release.

3. Remove the lid and press Cancel. Then choose Sauté low.

4. Stir in the ranch dressing, cream cheese, and cheddar jack cheese. Cook, stirring until well blended and warm.

Serving suggestion:

Serve with whole grain tortilla chips.

Exchange List Values

Meat—lean 1.5

Basic Nutritional Values

Calories 84 (Calories from Fat 108)
Total Fat 3 gm
(Saturated Fat 1.0 gm, Polyunsat Fat 0.2 gm, Monounsat Fat 0.5 gm)
Cholesterol 20 mg
Sodium 443 mg
Potassium 112 mg
Total Carb 2 gm
Dietary Fiber 0 gm
Sugars 1 gm
Protein 10 gm
Phosphorus 171 mg

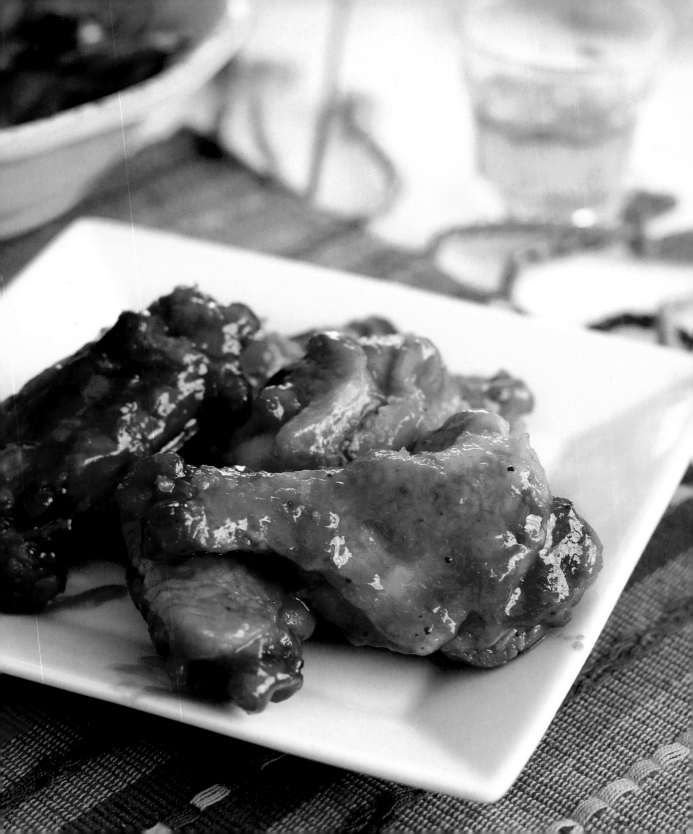

Levi's Sesame Chicken Wings

Shirley Unternahrer Hinh, Wayland, IA

Makes 16 appetizer servings
Prep. Time: 20 minutes & Cook Time: 13 minutes & Setting: Manual
Pressure: High & Release: Natural then Manual

1 cup water

3 pounds chicken wings

1 cup sugar substitute to equal 6 tablespoons sugar

¾ cup light soy sauce

½ cup no-salt-added ketchup

2 tablespoons canola oil

2 tablespoons sesame oil

2 garlic cloves, minced

Salt, to taste

Pepper, to taste

Toasted sesame seeds

1. Place the trivet in the Instant Pot inner pot with 1 cup of water. Carefully place the chicken wings on top of the trivet.

2. Seal the lid and make sure vent is set to sealing. Set the Instant Pot to Manual for 10 minutes.

3. While the wings are cooking, simmer the remaining ingredients, except the sesame seeds, in a small saucepan.

4. When cook time is up, let the pressure release naturally for 5 minutes, then perform a quick release of the remaining pressure.

5. Meanwhile, line a baking sheet with foil and place a baking rack on top. Turn the oven on to broil.

6. Carefully remove about half of the wings into a bowl and pour half of the sauce over the top. Gently stir to coat them, then place them on top of the baking rack. Repeat this process with the remaining wings and sauce.

7. Broil the wings about 5 inches from top of the oven for 5 minutes.

8. Sprinkle sesame seeds over top just before serving.

Exchange List Values

Carbohydrate 1.5
Meat—high fat 1.0

Basic Nutritional Values

Calories 192 (Calories from Fat 77)
Total Fat 9 gm
(Saturated Fat 1.8 gm, Polyunsat Fat 2.3 gm, Monounsat Fat 3.7 gm)

Cholesterol 22 mg
Sodium 453 mg
Total Carb 21 gm
Dietary Fiber 0 gm
Sugars 21 gm
Protein 9 gm

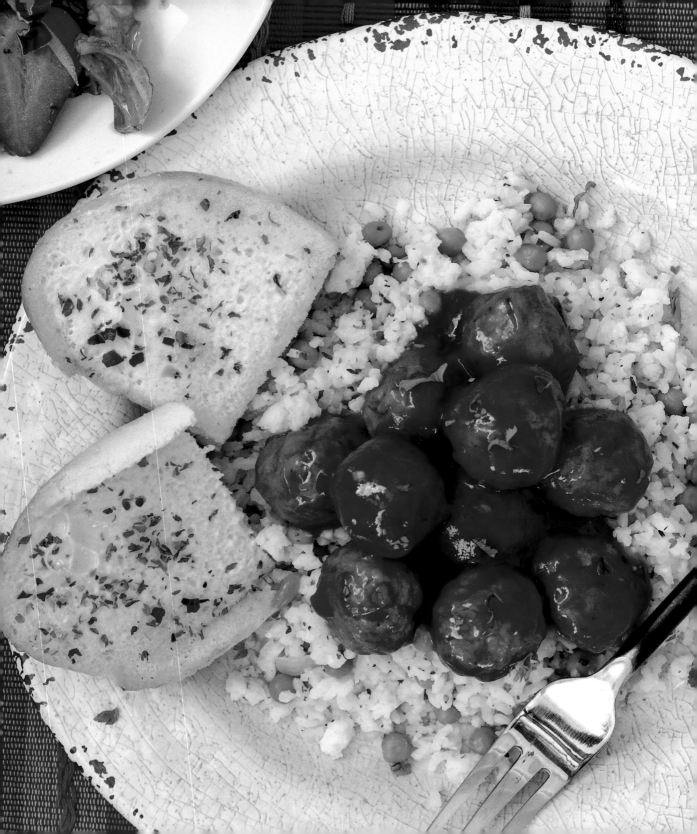

Smokey Barbecue Meatballs

Carla Koslowsky, Hillsboro, KS
Sherry Kreider, Lancaster, PA
Jennie Martin, Richfield, PA

Makes 10 servings, 1 meatball per serving
Prep. Time: 10 minutes ⚬ Cook Time: 19 minutes ⚬ Setting: Sauté then Manual
Pressure: High ⚬ Release: Manual

1½ pounds 90%-lean ground beef

½ cup quick oats

½ cup fat-free evaporated milk or milk

¼ cup egg substitute

¼–½ cup finely chopped onion, *optional*

¼ teaspoon garlic powder

¼ teaspoon pepper

¼ teaspoon chili powder

1 teaspoon salt

2 tablespoons olive oil

Sauce:

1½ cups ketchup

6 tablespoons Splenda Brown Sugar Blend

¼ cup chopped onion

¼ teaspoon liquid smoke

1. Mix ground beef, oats, milk, egg substitute, onion, garlic powder, pepper, chili powder, and salt together. Form 10 balls, each weighing about 2 ounces

2. Set the Instant Pot to Sauté and pour the olive oil into the inner pot. Once warm, add in the meatballs one at a time. Just try to make sure they're lightly browned on at least two sides. Turn the Instant Pot off by pressing Cancel.

3. Remove the meatballs onto a paper towel-lined plate and wipe the inner pot mostly clean of bits of meat and oil. Put the meatballs back into the inner pot.

4. Mix the sauce ingredients in a small bowl then pour them over the meatballs.

5. Secure the lid and make sure the vent is set to sealing. Cook on the Manual setting for 4 minutes.

6. When cooking time is up, perform a quick release of the pressure. Serve and enjoy!

Exchange List Values

Starch 1.0

Fat 2.5

Basic Nutritional Values

Calories 253 (Calories from Fat 90)

Total Fat 10 gm (Saturated Fat 3 gm, Polyunsat Fat 0.5 gm, Monounsat Fat 4.8 gm)

Cholesterol 44 mg

Sodium 592 mg

Potassium 349 mg

Total Carb 23 gm

Dietary Fiber 1 gm

Sugars 17 gm

Protein 16 gm

Phosphorus 138 mg

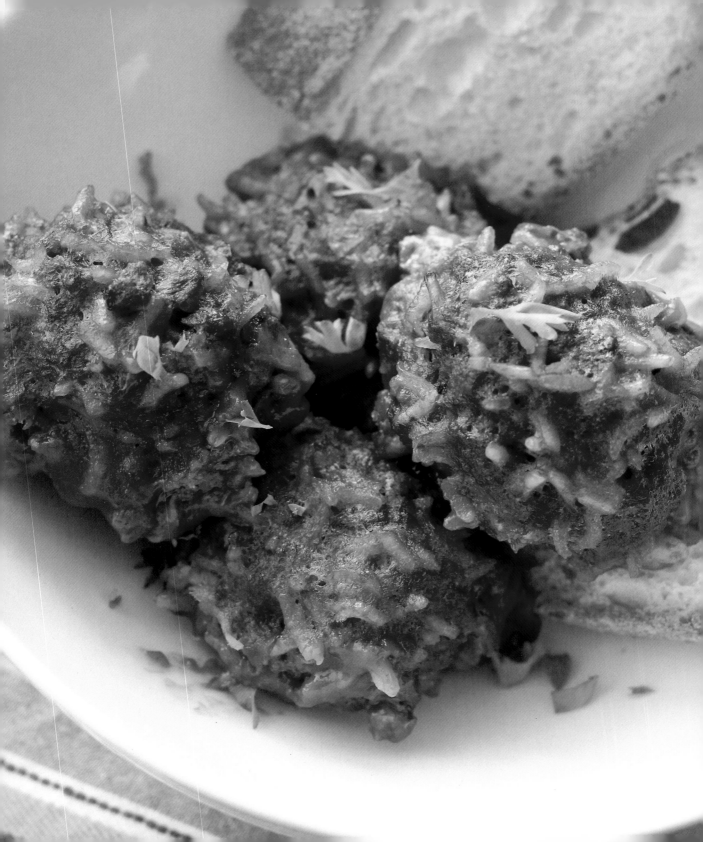

Porcupine Meatballs

Carolyn Spohn, Shawnee, KS

Makes about 8 meatballs
Prep. Time: 20 minutes   ♣   Cooking Time: 15 minutes   ♣   Setting: Meat
Pressure: High   ♣   Release: Natural

1 pound ground sirloin or turkey

½ cup raw brown rice, parboiled

1 egg

¼ cup finely minced onion

1 or 2 cloves garlic, minced

¼ teaspoon dried basil and/or oregano, *optional*

10¾-ounce can reduced-fat condensed tomato soup

½ soup can of water

1. Mix all ingredients, except tomato soup and water, in a bowl to combine well.

2. Form into balls about 1½-inch in diameter.

3. Mix tomato soup and water in the inner pot of the Instant Pot, then add the meatballs.

4. Secure the lid and make sure the vent is turned to sealing.

5. Press the Meat button and set for 15 minutes on high pressure.

6. Allow the pressure to release naturally after cook time is up.

Exchange List Values

Meat—very lean 2.0

Basic Nutritional Values

Calories 141 (Calories from Fat 18)
Total Fat 2 gm (Saturated Fat 0.7 gm, Polyunsat Fat 0.3 gm, Monounsat Fat 0.4 gm)
Cholesterol 50 mg
Sodium 176 mg
Potassium 262 mg
Total Carb 14 gm
Dietary Fiber 1 gm
Sugars 3 gm
Protein 16 gm
Phosphorus 50 mg

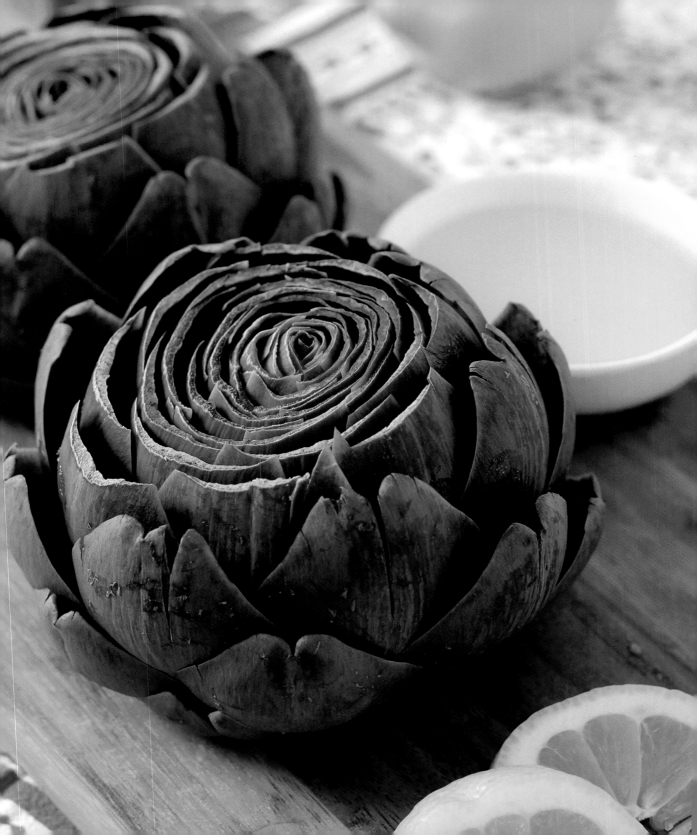

Artichokes

Susan Yoder Graber, Eureka, IL

Makes 4 servings
Prep. Time: 5 minutes ⚬ Cooking Time: 5–15 minutes ⚬ Setting: Manual
Pressure: High ⚬ Release: Manual

4 artichokes
1 cup water
2 tablespoons lemon juice
1 teaspoon salt

1. Wash and trim artichokes by cutting off the stems flush with the bottoms of the artichokes and by cutting ¾–1 inch off the tops. Stand upright in the bottom of the inner pot of the Instant Pot.

2. Pour water, lemon juice, and salt over artichokes.

3. Secure the lid and make sure the vent is set to sealing. On Manual, set the Instant Pot for 15 minutes for large artichokes, 10 minutes for medium artichokes, or 5 minutes for small artichokes.

4. When cook time is up, perform a quick release by releasing the pressure manually.

Serving suggestion:

Pull off individual leaves and dip bottom of each into melted margarine spread. Using your teeth, strip the individual leaf of the meaty portion at the bottom of each leaf. Or, dip the same way into light ranch dressing.

Exchange List Values

Vegetable 3.0

Basic Nutritional Values

Calories 60 (Calories from Fat 2)
Total Fat 0 gm
   (Saturated Fat 0.0 gm, Polyunsat Fat 0.1 gm, Monounsat Fat 0.0 gm)

Cholesterol 0 mg
Sodium 397 mg
Total Carb 13 gm
Dietary Fiber 6 gm
Sugars 1 gm
Protein 4 gm

Soups, Stews, Chilies & Chowders

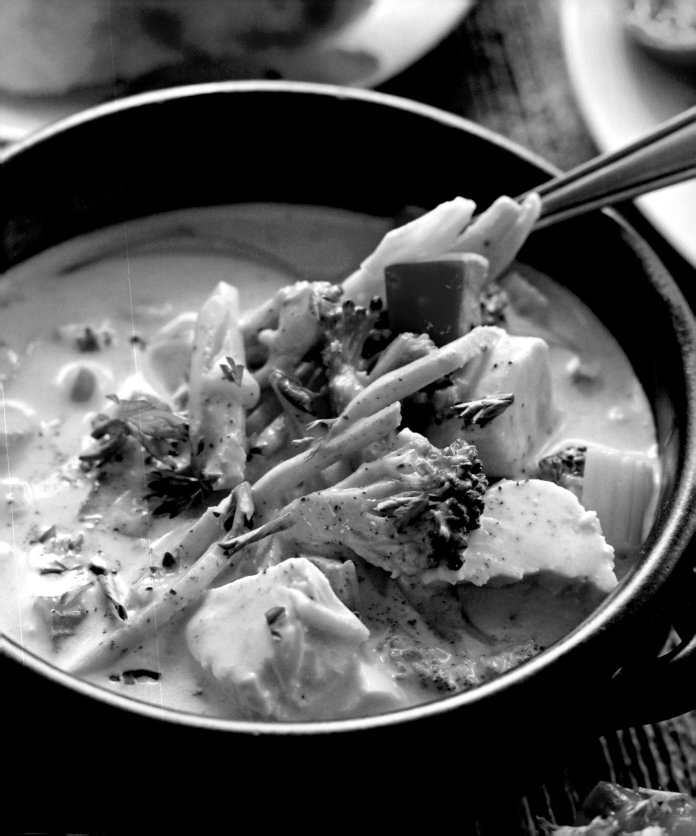

Chicken Cheddar Broccoli Soup

Maria Shevlin, Sicklerville, NJ

Makes 4–6 servings

Prep. Time: 15 minutes ⚬ Cooking Time: 15 minutes ⚬ Setting: Manual and Sauté
Pressure: High ⚬ Release: Manual

I pound raw chicken breast, thinly chopped/sliced

I pound fresh broccoli, chopped

½ cup onion, chopped

2 cloves garlic, minced

I cup shredded carrots

½ cup finely chopped celery

¼ cup finely chopped red bell pepper

3 cups low-sodium chicken bone broth

½ teaspoon salt

¼ teaspoon black pepper

½ teaspoon garlic powder

I teaspoon parsley flakes

Pinch red pepper flakes

2 cups evaporated skim milk

8 ounces freshly shredded low-fat cheddar cheese

2 tablespoons Frank's RedHot Original Cayenne Pepper Sauce

1. Place chicken, broccoli, onion, garlic, carrots, celery, bell pepper, chicken broth, and seasonings in the pot and stir to mix.

2. Secure the lid and make sure vent is at sealing. Place on Manual at high pressure for 15 minutes.

3. Manually release the pressure when cook time is up, remove lid, and stir in evaporated milk.

4. Place pot on Sauté setting until it all comes to a low boil, approximately 5 minutes.

5. Stir in cheese and the hot sauce.

6. Turn off the pot as soon as you add the cheese and give it a stir.

7. Continue to stir till the cheese is melted.

Serving suggestion:

Serve it up with slice or two of whole grain bread.

Exchange List Values

Starch 2.0

Fat 0.0

Meat—lean 4.5

Vegetable 1.5

Basic Nutritional Values

Calories 302 (Calories from Fat 54)

Total Fat 6 gm (Saturated Fat 2.6 gm, Polyunsat Fat 0.7 gm, Monounsat Fat 1.7 gm)

Cholesterol 73 mg

Sodium 753 mg

Total Carb 20 gm

Dietary Fiber 3 gm

Sugars 14 gm

Protein 41 gm

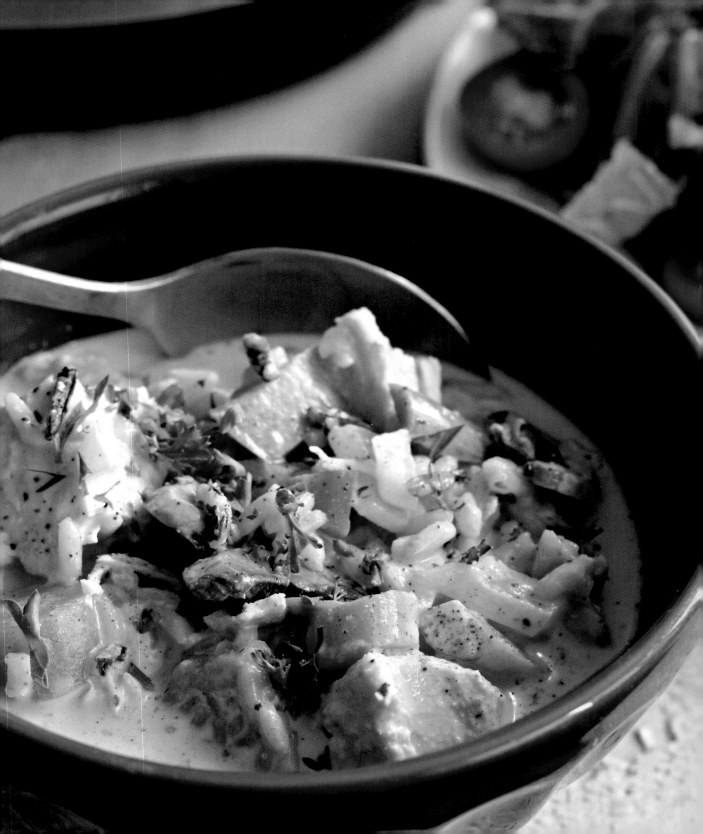

Creamy Chicken Wild Rice Soup

Vonnie Oyer, Hubbard, OR

Makes 4–6 servings
Prep. Time: 15 minutes ⚭ *Cooking Time: 15 minutes* ⚭ *Setting: Sauté and Manual*
Pressure: High ⚭ *Release: Manual*

2 tablespoons margarine

½ cup yellow onion, diced

¾ cup carrots, diced

¾ cup sliced mushrooms
(about 3–4 mushrooms)

½ pound chicken breast, diced
into 1-inch cubes

6.2-ounce box Uncle Ben's Long Grain
& Wild Rice Fast Cook

2 14-ounce cans low-sodium
chicken broth

1 cup skim milk

1 cup evaporated skim milk

2 ounces fat-free cream cheese

2 tablespoons cornstarch

1. Select the Sauté feature and add the margarine, onion, carrots, and mushrooms to the inner pot. Sauté for about 5 minutes until onions are translucent and soft.

2. Add the cubed chicken and seasoning packet from the Uncle Ben's box and stir to combine.

3. Add the rice and chicken broth. Select Manual, high pressure, then lock the lid and make sure the vent is set to sealing. Set the time for 5 minutes.

4. After the cooking time ends, allow it to stay on Keep Warm for 5 minutes and then quick release the pressure.

5. Remove the lid; change the setting to the Sauté function again.

6. Add the skim milk, evaporated milk, and cream cheese. Stir to melt.

7. In a small bowl, mix the cornstarch with a little bit of water to dissolve, then add to the soup to thicken.

Exchange List Values	Basic Nutritional Values	
Starch 4.0	Calories 316 (Calories from Fat 54)	Cholesterol 59 mg
Fat 0.5		Sodium 638 mg
Meat—lean 1.5	Total Fat 7 gm	Total Carb 35 gm
Vegetable 2.5	(Saturated Fat 1.5 gm, Polyunsat Fat 1.5 gm, Monounsat Fat 2.4 gm)	Dietary Fiber 1 gm
		Sugars 10 gm
		Protein 27 gm

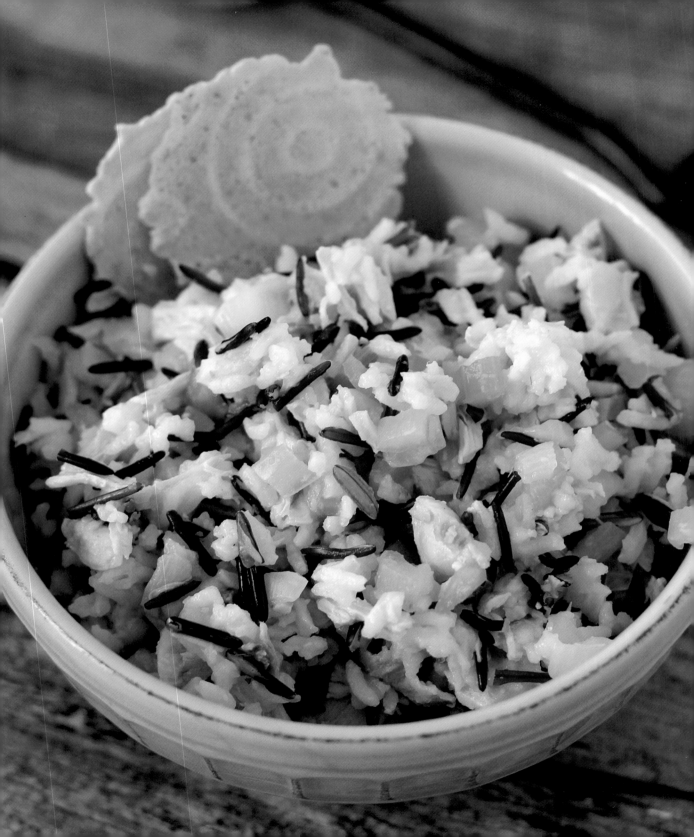

Chicken Rice Soup

Karen Ceneviva, Seymour, CT

Makes 8 servings
Prep Time: 10 minutes ⚭ Cooking Time: 10 minutes ⚭ Setting: Sauté and Manual
Pressure: High ⚭ Release: Natural then Manual

1 teaspoon vegetable oil

2 ribs celery, chopped in ½"-thick pieces

1 medium onion, chopped

1 cup wild rice, uncooked

½ cup long-grain rice, uncooked

1 pound boneless skinless chicken breasts, cut into ¾" cubes

5¼ cups fat-free, low-sodium chicken broth

2 teaspoons dried thyme leaves

¼ teaspoon red pepper flakes

1. Using the Sauté function on the Instant Pot, heat the teaspoon of vegetable oil. Sauté the celery and onion until the onions are slightly translucent (3–5 minutes). Once cooked, press Cancel.

2. Add the remaining ingredients to the inner pot.

3. Secure the lid and make sure the vent is set to sealing. Using the Manual function, set the time to 10 minutes.

4. When cook time is over, let the pressure release naturally for 10 minutes, then perform a quick release.

Serving suggestion:
A dollop of fat-free sour cream sprinkled with finely chopped scallions on top of each individual serving bowl makes a nice finishing touch.

Exchange List Values

Starch 1.0
Meat—lean 2.0

Basic Nutritional Values

Calories 160 (Calories from Fat 20)
Total Fat 2 gm (Saturated Fat 0 gm, Polyunsat Fat 0.5 gm, Monounsat Fat 1.0 gm)

Cholesterol 35 mg
Sodium 375 mg
Total Carb 18 gm
Dietary Fiber 1 gm
Sugars 2 gm
Protein 16 gm

Chicken Vegetable Soup

Maria Shevlin, Sicklerville, NJ

Makes 6 servings
Prep. Time: 12–25 minutes ⚜ Cooking Time: 4 minutes ⚜ Setting: Manual
Pressure: High ⚜ Release: Manual

1–2 raw chicken breasts, cubed
½ medium onion, chopped
4 cloves garlic, minced
½ sweet potato, small cubes
1 large carrot, peeled and cubed
4 stalks celery, chopped, leaves included
½ cup frozen corn
¼ cup frozen peas
¼ cup frozen lima beans
1 cup frozen green beans (bite-sized)
¼–½ cup chopped savoy cabbage
14½-ounce can low-sodium petite diced tomatoes
3 cups low-sodium chicken bone broth
½ teaspoon black pepper
1 teaspoon garlic powder
¼ cup chopped fresh parsley
¼–½ teaspoon red pepper flakes

1. Add all of the ingredients, in the order listed, to the inner pot of the Instant Pot.

2. Lock the lid in place, set the vent to sealing, press Manual, and cook at high pressure for 4 minutes.

3. Release the pressure manually as soon as cooking time is finished.

Exchange List Values

Starch 2.0
Fat 0.0
Meat—very lean 2.0
Vegetable 1.0

Basic Nutritional Values

Calories 176 (Calories from Fat 23)
Total Fat 3 gm (Saturated Fat 0.6 gm, Polyunsat Fat 0.5 gm, Monounsat Fat 0.6 gm)
Cholesterol 56 mg
Sodium 169 mg
Total Carb 18 gm
Dietary Fiber 4 gm
Sugars 7 gm
Protein 21 gm

Nancy's Vegetable Beef Soup

Nancy Graves, Manhattan, KS

Makes 8 servings

Prep. Time: 25 minutes & Cooking Time: 8 hours & Setting: Slow Cook

2-pound roast, cubed, or 2 pounds stewing meat

15-ounce can corn

15-ounce can green beans

1-pound bag frozen peas

40-ounce can no-added-salt stewed tomatoes

5 teaspoons salt-free beef bouillon powder

Tabasco, to taste

½ teaspoons salt

1. Combine all ingredients in the Instant Pot. Do not drain vegetables.

2. Add water to fill inner pot only to the fill line.

3. Secure the lid, or use the glass lid and set the Instant Pot on Slow Cook mode, Low for 8 hours, or until meat is tender and vegetables are soft.

Exchange List Values

Starch 1.0
Vegetable 2.0
Meat—lean 2.0

Basic Nutritional Values

Calories 229 (Calories from Fat 46)
Total Fat 5 gm
(Saturated Fat 1.4 gm, Polyunsat Fat 0.5 gm, Monounsat Fat 2.2 gm)

Cholesterol 56 mg
Sodium 545 mg
Total Carb 24 gm
Dietary Fiber 6 gm
Sugars 10 gm
Protein 23 gm

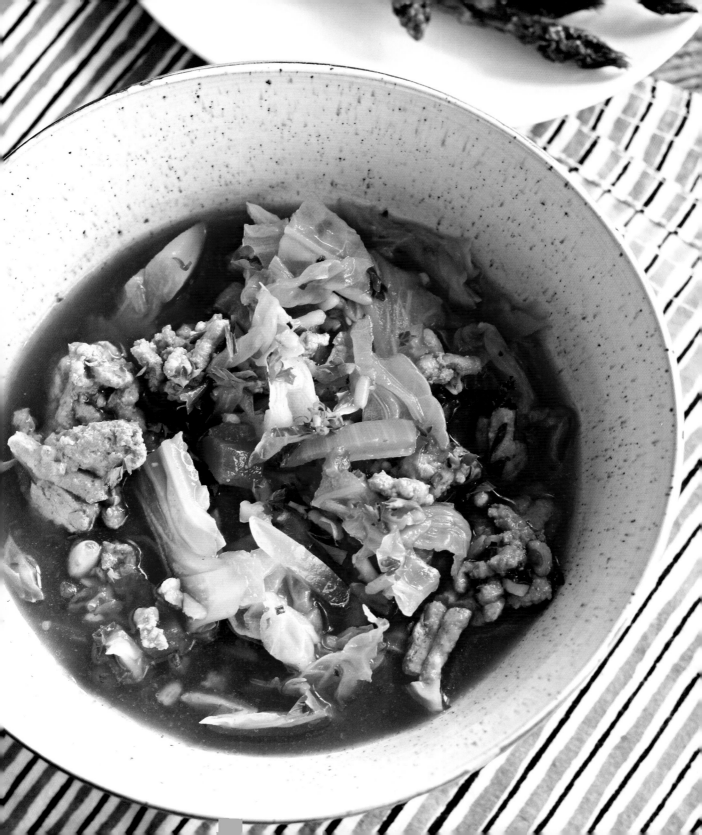

Unstuffed Cabbage Soup

Colleen Heatwole, Burton, MI

Makes 4–6 servings
Prep. Time: 15 minutes ⚜ Cooking Time: 20 minutes ⚜ Setting: Sauté and Manual
Pressure: High ⚜ Release: Natural then Manual

2 tablespoons coconut oil

1 pound ground sirloin or turkey

1 medium onion, diced

2 cloves garlic, minced

1 small head cabbage, chopped, cored, cut into roughly 2-inch pieces.

6-ounce can low-sodium tomato paste

32-ounce can low-sodium diced tomatoes, with liquid

2 cups low-sodium beef broth

1½ cups water

¾ cup brown rice

1–2 teaspoons salt

½ teaspoon black pepper

1 teaspoon oregano

1 teaspoon parsley

1. Melt coconut oil in the inner pot of the Instant Pot using Sauté function. Add ground meat. Stir frequently until meat loses color, about 2 minutes.

2. Add onion and garlic and continue to sauté for 2 more minutes, stirring frequently.

3. Add chopped cabbage.

4. On top of cabbage layer tomato paste, tomatoes with liquid, beef broth, water, rice, and spices.

5. Secure the lid and set vent to sealing. Using Manual setting, select 20 minutes.

6. When time is up, let the pressure release naturally for 10 minutes, then do a quick release.

Exchange List Values

Starch 3.5

Fat 0.5

Meat—lean 1.0

Vegetable 2.0

Basic Nutritional Values

Calories 282 (Calories from Fat 54)

Total Fat 6 gm
(Saturated Fat 4.2 gm, Polyunsat Fat 0.4 gm, Monounsat Fat 0.6 gm)

Cholesterol 37 mg

Sodium 898 mg

Total Carb 34 gm

Dietary Fiber 3 gm

Sugars 6 gm

Protein 23 gm

Beef Dumpling Soup

Barbara Walker, Sturgis, SD

Makes 6 servings
Prep. Time: 35 minutes ⚭ Cooking Time: 6½ hours ⚭ Setting: Slow Cook

1 pound beef stewing meat, trimmed of visible fat, cubed

1 recipe onion soup mix, dry, salt-free

6 cups water

2 carrots, shredded

1 celery rib, finely chopped

1 tomato, peeled and chopped

2 cloves garlic

½ teaspoon dried basil

¼ teaspoon dill weed

1 cup buttermilk biscuit mix

1 tablespoon finely chopped parsley

6 tablespoons fat-free milk

1. Place meat in inner pot of the Instant Pot. Sprinkle with onion soup mix. Pour water over meat.

2. Add carrots, celery, tomato, garlic, basil and dill weed.

3. Secure the lid, or cover with the glass lid. Cook on the Slow Cook setting, Low, for 6 hours, or until meat is tender.

4. Combine biscuit mix and parsley. Stir in milk with fork until moistened. Drop dumplings by teaspoonfuls into pot.

5. Secure the lid once more, then cook on high Slow Cook mode for 30 minutes more.

Exchange List Values

Starch 1.0
Vegetable 1.0
Meat—lean 1.0
Fat 0.5

Basic Nutritional Values

Calories 206 (Calories from Fat 57)
Total Fat 6 gm
(Saturated Fat 0.9 gm, Polyunsat Fat 1.4 gm, Monounsat Fat 2.6 gm)

Cholesterol 38 mg
Sodium 329 mg
Total Carb 22 gm
Dietary Fiber 2 gm
Sugars 6 gm
Protein 15 gm

French Market Soup

Ethel Mumaw, Berlin, OH

Makes 8 servings (about 2½ quarts total)
Prep. Time: 20 minutes ⚜ Cooking Time: 1 hour ⚜ Setting: Manual
Pressure: High ⚜ Release: Natural

2 cups mixed dry beans, washed with stones removed

7 cups water

I ham hock, all visible fat removed

I teaspoon salt

¼ teaspoon pepper

16-ounce can low-sodium tomatoes

I large onion, chopped

I garlic clove, minced

I chile, chopped, or
I teaspoon chili powder

¼ cup lemon juice

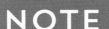

1. Combine all ingredients in the inner pot of the Instant Pot.

2. Secure the lid and make sure vent is set to sealing. Using Manual, set the Instant Pot to cook for 60 minutes.

3. When cooking time is over, let the pressure release naturally. When the Instant Pot is ready, unlock the lid, then remove the bone and any hard or fatty pieces. Pull the meat off the bone and chop into small pieces. Add the ham back into the Instant Pot.

NOTE

If you want your soup to be a little thicker, mash the beans a bit and it will naturally thicken up.

Exchange List Values

Starch 1.5
Vegetable 1.0
Meat—lean 1.0

Basic Nutritional Values

Calories 191 (Calories from Fat 34)
Total Fat 4 gm
(Saturated Fat 1.3 gm, Polyunsat Fat 0.6 gm, Monounsat Fat 1.5 gm)

Cholesterol 9 mg
Sodium 488 mg
Total Carb 29 gm
Dietary Fiber 7 gm
Sugars 5 gm
Protein 12 gm

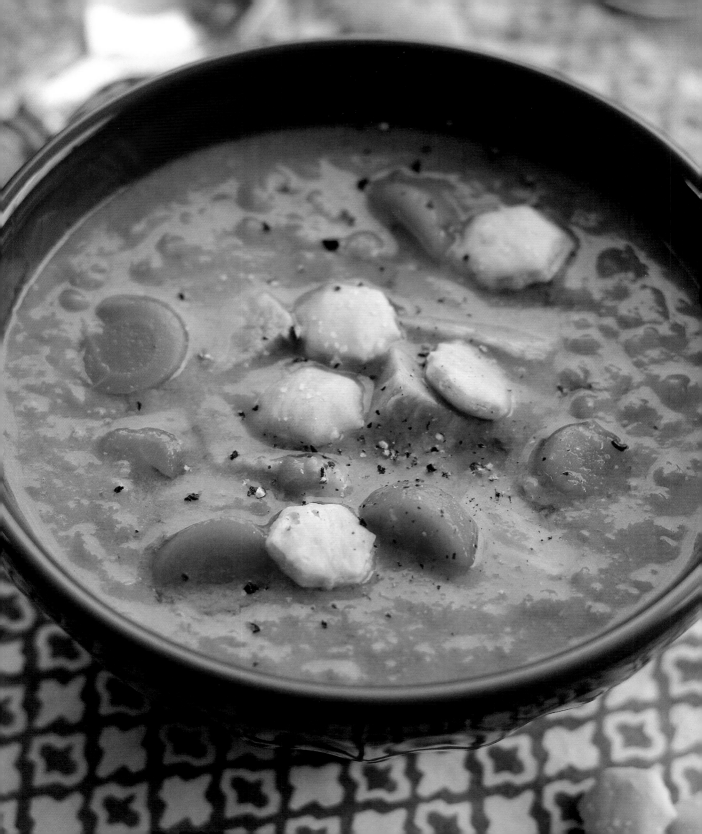

Split Pea Soup

Judy Gascho, Woodburn, OR

Makes 3–4 servings
Prep. Time: 20 minutes ⚜ Cooking Time: 15 minutes ⚜ Setting: Manual
Pressure: High ⚜ Release: Manual

4 cups low-sodium chicken broth

4 sprigs thyme

4 ounces ham, diced (about ⅓ cup)

2 tablespoons margarine

2 stalks celery

2 carrots

1 large leek

3 cloves garlic

1½ cups dried green split peas (about 12 ounces)

Salt and pepper to taste

1. Pour the broth into the inner pot of the Instant Pot and set to Sauté. Add the thyme, ham, and margarine.

2. While the broth heats, chop the celery and cut the carrots into ½-inch-thick rounds. Halve the leek lengthwise and thinly slice and chop the garlic. Add the vegetables to the pot as you cut them. Rinse the split peas in a colander, discarding any stones, then add to the pot.

3. Secure the lid, making sure the steam valve is in the sealing position. Set the cooker to Manual at high pressure for 15 minutes. When the time is up, carefully turn the steam valve to the venting position to release the pressure manually.

4. Turn off the Instant Pot. Remove the lid and stir the soup; discard the thyme sprigs.

5. Thin the soup with up to one cup water if needed (the soup will continue to thicken as it cools). Season with salt and pepper.

Exchange List Values

Starch 2.0
Fat 1.5
Meat—medium 0.5
Vegetable 1.5

Basic Nutritional Values

Calories 200 (Calories from Fat 81)
Total Fat 9 gm
(Saturated Fat 2.1 gm, Polyunsat Fat 2.2 gm, Monounsat Fat 3.9 gm)

Cholesterol 19 mg
Sodium 450 mg
Total Carb 20 gm
Dietary Fiber 2 gm
Sugars 3 gm
Protein 12 gm

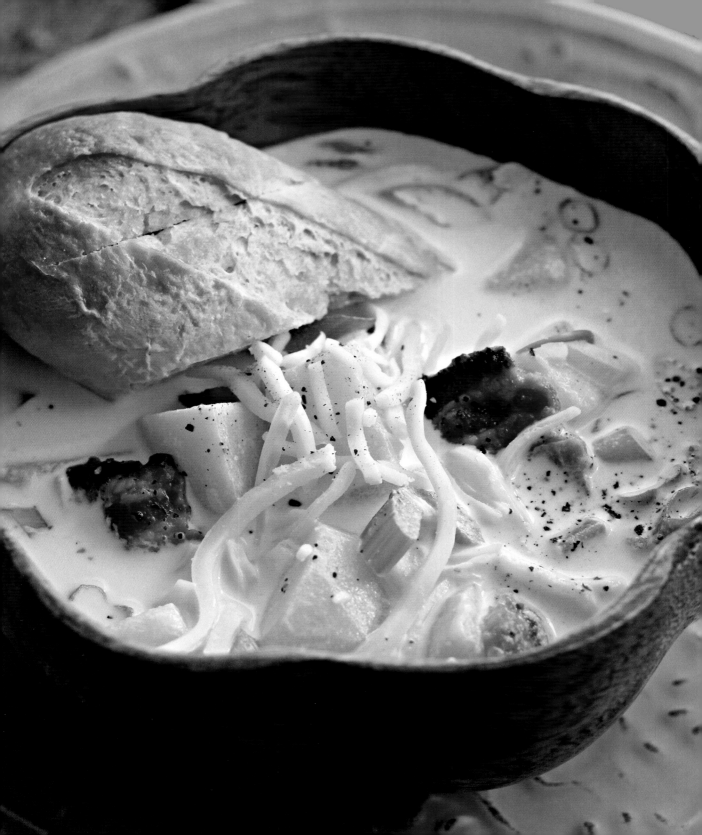

Potato Bacon Soup

Colleen Heatwole, Burton, MI

Makes 4–6 servings
Prep. Time: 30 minutes ⚭ Cooking Time: 5 minutes ⚭ Setting: Manual
Pressure: High ⚭ Release: Manual

5 pounds potatoes, peeled and cubed

3 stalks of celery, diced into roughly ¼- to ½-inch pieces

1 large onion, chopped

1 clove garlic, minced

½ teaspoon black pepper

4 cups low-sodium chicken broth

1 pound bacon, fried crisp and rough chopped

1 cup evaporated skim milk

1 cup skim milk

Salt to taste

Low-fat sour cream, reduced-fat shredded cheddar cheese, and diced green onion to garnish, *optional*

1. Place potatoes in bottom of the Instant Pot inner pot.

2. Add celery, onion, garlic, and pepper, then stir to combine.

3. Add chicken broth and bacon to pot and stir to combine.

4. Secure the lid and make sure vent is in the sealing position. Using Manual mode, select 5 minutes, high pressure.

5. Manually release the pressure when cooking time is up. Open pot and roughly mash potatoes, leaving some large chunks if desired.

6. Add evaporated skim milk and skim milk.

7. Serve while still hot with desired amount of salt and assortment of garnishes.

Exchange List Values

Starch 8.0
Fat 5.5
Meat—medium 1.0
Vegetable 45

Basic Nutritional Values

Calories 735 (Calories from Fat 288)
Total Fat 32 gm (Saturated Fat 10.7 gm, Polyunsat Fat 3.6 gm, Monounsat Fat 14 gm)

Cholesterol 85 mg
Sodium 1932 mg
Total Carb 70 gm
Dietary Fiber 10 gm
Sugars 13 gm
Protein 40 gm

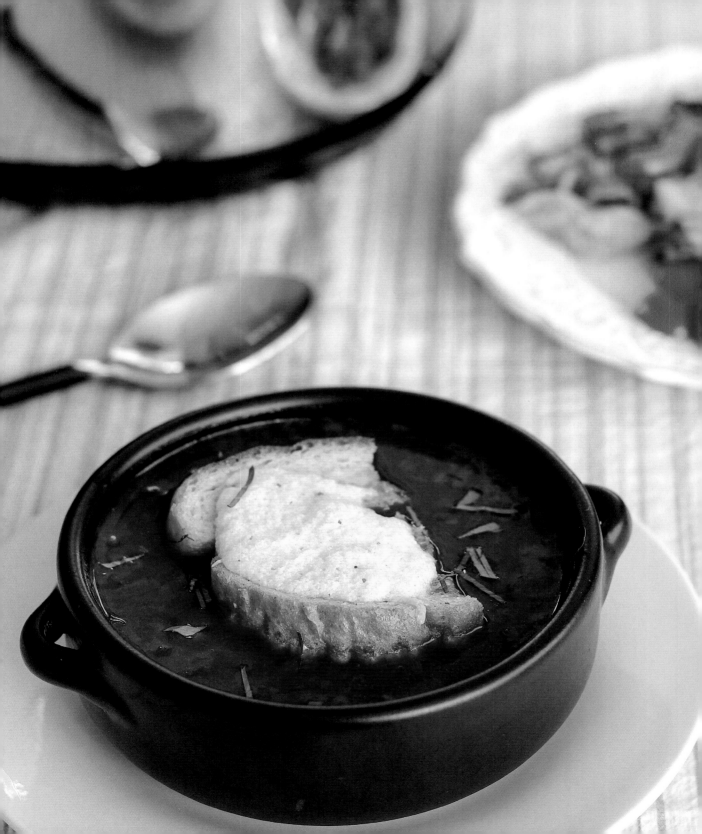

French Onion Soup

Jenny R. Unternahrer, Wayland, IA
Janice Yoskovich, Carmichaels, PA

Makes 10 servings
Prep. Time: 10 minutes ⚘ Cooking Time: 20 minutes ⚘ Setting: Sauté and Manual
Pressure: High ⚘ Release: Natural then Manual

½ cup light, soft tub margarine

8–10 large onions, sliced

3 14-ounce cans 98% fat-free, lower-sodium beef broth

2½ cups water

3 teaspoons sodium-free chicken bouillon powder

1½ teaspoons Worcestershire sauce

3 bay leaves

10 (1-ounce) slices French bread, toasted

1. Turn the Instant Pot to the Sauté function and add in the margarine and onions. Cook about 5 minutes, or until the onions are slightly soft. Press Cancel.

2. Add the beef broth, water, bouillon powder, Worcestershire sauce, and bay leaves and stir.

3. Secure the lid and make sure vent is set to sealing. Cook on Manual mode for 20 minutes.

4. Let the pressure release naturally for 15 minutes, then do a quick release. Open the lid and discard bay leaves.

5. Ladle into bowls. Top each with a slice of bread and some cheese if you desire.

Exchange List Values

Starch 1.0
Vegetable 3.0
Fat 0.5

Basic Nutritional Values

Calories 178 (Calories from Fat 35)
Total Fat 4 gm
(Saturated Fat 0.3 gm, Polyunsat Fat 0.9 gm, Monounsat Fat 2.0 gm)

Cholesterol 0 mg
Sodium 476 mg
Total Carb 31 gm
Dietary Fiber 4 gm
Sugars 12 gm
Protein 6 gm

Italian Vegetable Soup

Patti Boston, Newark, OH

Makes 6 servings

Prep. Time: 20 minutes ⚘ *Cooking Time: 4¾–9¼ hours* ⚘ *Setting: Slow Cook*

3 small carrots, sliced

1 small onion, chopped

2 small potatoes, diced

2 tablespoons chopped parsley

1 garlic clove, minced

3 teaspoons sodium-free beef bouillon powder

1¼ teaspoons dried basil

¼ teaspoon pepper

16-ounce can red kidney beans, undrained

3 cups water

14½-ounce can stewed tomatoes, with juice

1 cup diced, extra-lean, lower-sodium cooked ham

1. In the inner pot of the Instant Pot, layer the carrots, onion, potatoes, parsley, garlic, beef bouillon, basil, pepper, and kidney beans. Do not stir. Add water.

2. Secure the lid and cook on the Low Slow Cook mode for 8–9 hours, or on high 4½–5½ hours, until vegetables are tender.

3. Remove the lid and stir in the tomatoes and ham. Secure the lid again and cook on high Slow Cook mode for 10–15 minutes more.

Exchange List Values

Starch 1.5

Vegetable 2.0

Basic Nutritional Values

Calories 156 (Calories from Fat 7)

Total Fat 1 gm (Saturated Fat 0.2 gm, Polyunsat Fat 0.3 gm, Monounsat Fat 0.2 gm)

Cholesterol 9 mg

Sodium 614 mg

Total Carb 29 gm

Dietary Fiber 5 gm

Sugars 8 gm

Protein 9 gm

Pork Chili

Carol Duree, Salina, KS

Makes 5 servings

Prep. Time: 15 minutes ⚜ *Cooking Time: 4–8 hours* ⚜ *Setting: Slow Cook*

1 pound boneless pork ribs

2 14½-ounce cans fire-roasted diced tomatoes

4¼-ounce cans diced green chiles, drained

½ cup chopped onion

1 clove garlic, minced

1 tablespoon chili powder

1. Layer the ingredients into the Instant Pot inner pot in the order given.

2. Secure the lid. Cook on the high Slow Cook function for 4 hours or on low 6–8 hours, or until pork is tender but not dry.

3. Cut up or shred meat. Stir into the chili and serve.

NOTES

1. You can serve this as soup, but we especially like it over brown rice.

2. You can add a 1-pound can of your favorite chili beans 30 minutes before end of cooking time.

Exchange List Values

Vegetable 2.0
Meat—lean 2.0
Fat 1.0

Basic Nutritional Values

Calories 180 (Calories from Fat 65)
Total Fat 7 gm
   (Saturated Fat 2.5 gm, Polyunsat Fat 1.0 gm, Monounsat Fat 3.0 gm)

Cholesterol 55 mg
Sodium 495 mg
Total Carb 12 gm
Dietary Fiber 3 gm
Sugars 6 gm
Protein 18 gm

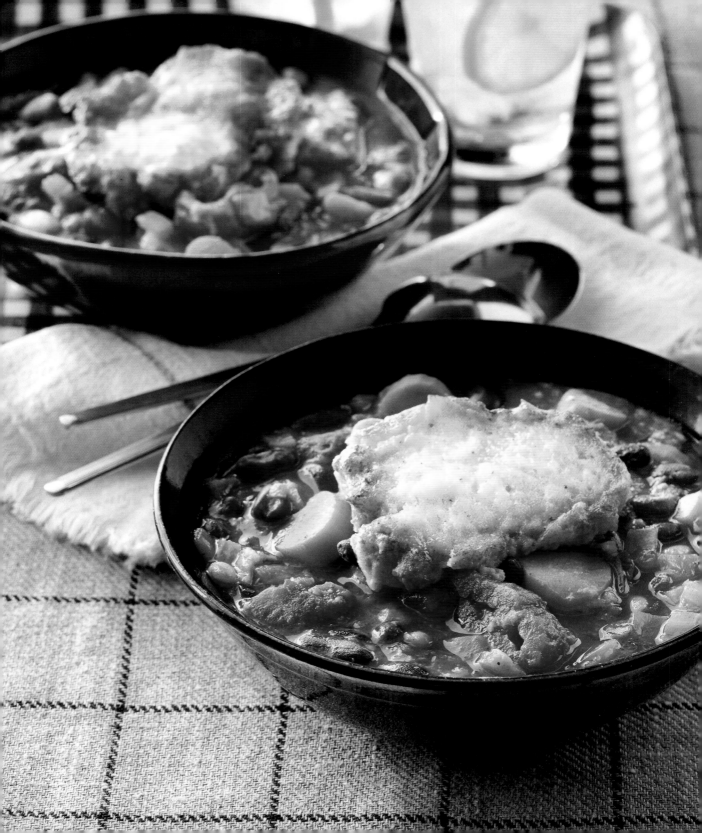

Southwestern Bean Soup with Corn Dumplings

Melba Eshleman, Manheim, PA

Makes 8 servings

Prep. Time: 50 minutes ⚜ *Cooking Time: 4½–12½ hours* ⚜ *Setting: Slow Cook*

15½-ounce can red kidney beans, rinsed and drained

15½-ounce can black beans, pinto beans, or great northern beans, rinsed and drained

3 cups water

14½-ounce can Mexican-style stewed tomatoes

10-ounce package frozen whole-kernel corn, thawed

1 cup sliced carrots

1 cup chopped onions

4-ounce can chopped green chilies

3 teaspoons sodium-free instant bouillon powder (any flavor)

1–2 teaspoons chili powder

2 cloves garlic, minced

Dumplings:

⅓ cup flour

¼ cup yellow cornmeal

1 teaspoon baking powder

Dash of pepper

1 egg white, beaten

2 tablespoons milk

1 tablespoon oil

1. Combine the 11 soup ingredients in inner pot of the Instant Pot.

2. Secure the lid and cook on the Low Slow Cook setting for 10–12 hours or high for 4–5 hours.

3. Make dumplings by mixing together flour, cornmeal, baking powder, and pepper.

4. Combine egg white, milk, and oil. Add to flour mixture. Stir with fork until just combined.

5. At the end of the soup's cooking time, turn the Instant Pot to Slow Cook function high if you don't already have it there. Remove the lid and drop dumpling mixture by rounded teaspoonfuls to make 8 mounds atop the soup.

6. Secure the lid once more and cook for an additional 30 minutes.

Exchange List Values

Starch 2.0

Vegetable 2.0

Basic Nutritional Values

Calories 197 (Calories from Fat 13)

Total Fat 1 gm (Saturated Fat 0.2 gm, Polyunsat Fat 0.6 gm, Monounsat Fat 0.5 gm)

Cholesterol 0 mg

Sodium 367 mg

Total Carb 39 gm

Dietary Fiber 8 gm

Sugars 6 gm

Protein 9 gm

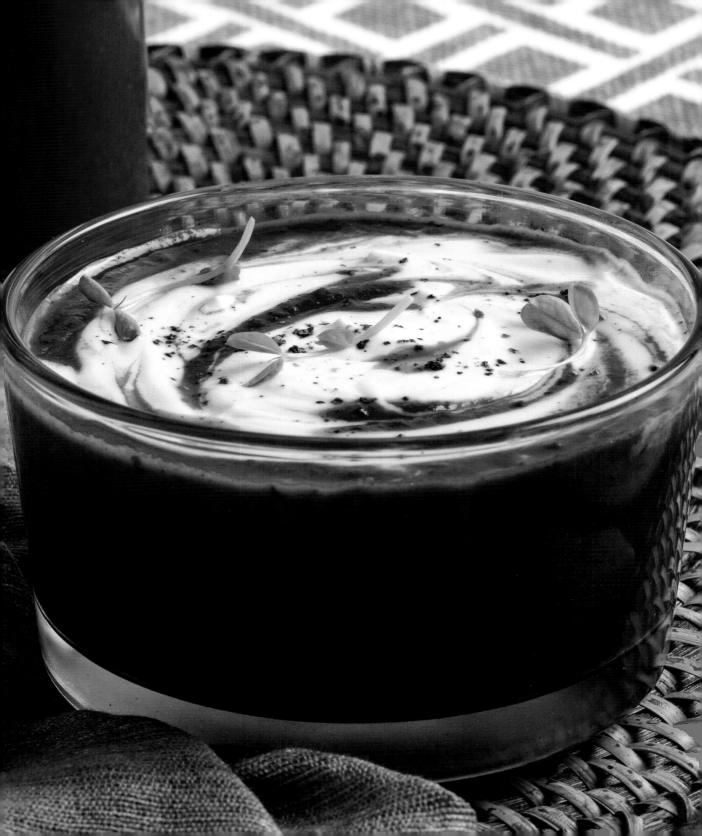

Black Bean Soup

Colleen Heatwole, Burton, MI

Makes 4 servings

Prep. Time: 20 minutes ⚜ Cooking Time: 25 minutes (unless beans have been soaked) ⚜ Setting: Sauté and Bean/Chili ⚜ Pressure: High ⚜ Release: Natural

2 tablespoons coconut oil

1 cup coarsely chopped onion

2 cups dry black beans, cleaned of debris and rinsed

6 cups low-sodium vegetable or chicken broth

3 cloves garlic, minced

½ teaspoon paprika

⅛ teaspoon red pepper flakes

2 large bay leaves

1 teaspoon cumin

2 teaspoons oregano

½ teaspoon salt (more if desired)

Nonfat yogurt, nonfat sour cream for garnish, *optional*

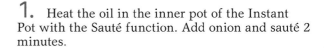

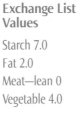

1. Heat the oil in the inner pot of the Instant Pot with the Sauté function. Add onion and sauté 2 minutes.

2. Add remaining ingredients except garnishes, and stir well.

3. Secure lid and make sure vent is at sealing, then set to Bean/Chili for 25 minutes.

4. After time is up let pressure release naturally.

5. Remove lid, then remove the bay leaves and serve with desired garnishes.

Exchange List Values

Starch 7.0

Fat 2.0

Meat—lean 0

Vegetable 4.0

Basic Nutritional Values

Calories 428 (Calories from Fat 81)

Total Fat 9 gm (Saturated Fat 6.3 gm, Polyunsat Fat 0.9 gm, Monounsat Fat 0.6 gm)

Cholesterol 3 mg

Sodium 335 mg

Total Carb 64 gm

Dietary Fiber 16 gm

Sugars 4 gm

Protein 23 gm

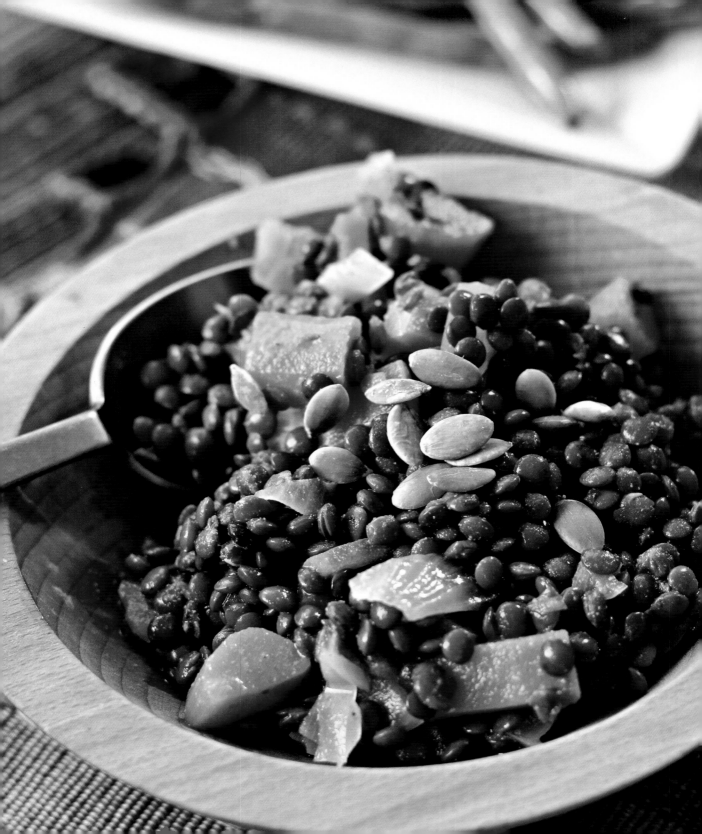

Brown Lentil Soup

Colleen Heatwole, Burton, MI

Makes 3–5 servings
Prep. Time: 15 minutes ⚹ *Cooking Time: 20 minutes* ⚹ *Setting: Sauté and Manual*
Pressure: High ⚹ *Release: Manual*

1 medium onion, chopped

1 tablespoon olive oil

1 medium carrot, diced

2 cloves garlic, minced

1 small bay leaf

1 pound brown lentils

5 cups low-sodium chicken broth

¼ teaspoon ground black pepper

½ teaspoon lemon juice

1. Using the Sauté function, sauté the chopped onion in oil in the inner pot of the Instant Pot about 2 minutes, or until it starts to soften.

2. Add diced carrot and sauté 3 minutes more until it begins to soften. Stir frequently or it will stick.

3. Add garlic and sauté 1 more minute.

4. Add bay leaf, lentils, and broth to pot.

5. Secure the lid and make sure vent is at sealing. Using Manual setting, select 14 minutes and cook on high pressure.

6. When cooking time is up, do a quick release of the pressure.

7. Discard bay leaf.

8. Stir in pepper and lemon juice, then adjust seasonings to taste.

Exchange List Values

Starch 0.5

Fat 0.0

Meat—lean 1.0

Vegetable 0.5

Basic Nutritional Values

Calories 151 (Calories from Fat 27)

Total Fat 4 gm (Saturated Fat 0.7 gm, Polyunsat Fat 0.6 gm, Monounsat Fat 2.1 gm)

Cholesterol 2 mg

Sodium 79 mg

Total Carb 5 gm

Dietary Fiber 1 gm

Sugars 3 gm

Protein 10 gm

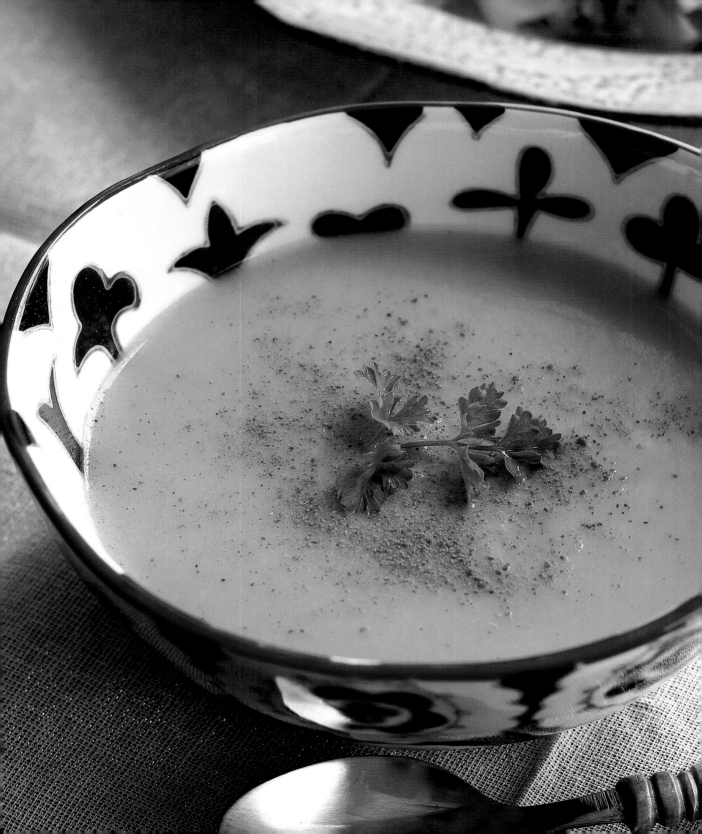

Butternut Squash Soup

Colleen Heatwole, Burton, MI

Makes 4 servings
Prep. Time: 30 minutes ⚜ Cooking Time: 15 minutes ⚜ Setting: Sauté and Manual
Pressure: High ⚜ Release: Manual

2 tablespoons margarine

1 large onion, chopped

2 cloves garlic, minced

1 teaspoon thyme

½ teaspoon sage

Salt and pepper to taste

2 large butternut squash, peeled, seeded, and cubed (about 4 pounds)

4 cups low-sodium chicken stock

1. In the inner pot of the Instant Pot, melt the margarine using Sauté function.

2. Add onion and garlic and cook until soft, 3 to 5 minutes.

3. Add thyme and sage and cook another minute. Season with salt and pepper.

4. Stir in butternut squash and add chicken stock.

5. Secure the lid and make sure vent is at sealing. Using Manual setting, cook squash and seasonings 10 minutes, using high pressure.

6. When time is up, do a quick release of the pressure.

7. Puree the soup in a food processor or use immersion blender right in the inner pot. If soup is too thick, add more stock. Adjust salt and pepper as needed.

Exchange List Values

Starch 6.0

Fat 1.5

Meat—medium 0

Vegetable 4.0

Basic Nutritional Values

Calories 279 (Calories from Fat 59)

Total Fat 7 gm (Saturated Fat 1.4 gm, Polyunsat Fat 1.9 gm, Monounsat Fat 2.7 gm)

Cholesterol 2 mg

Sodium 144 mg

Total Carb 56 gm

Dietary Fiber 9 gm

Sugars 11 gm

Protein 6 gm

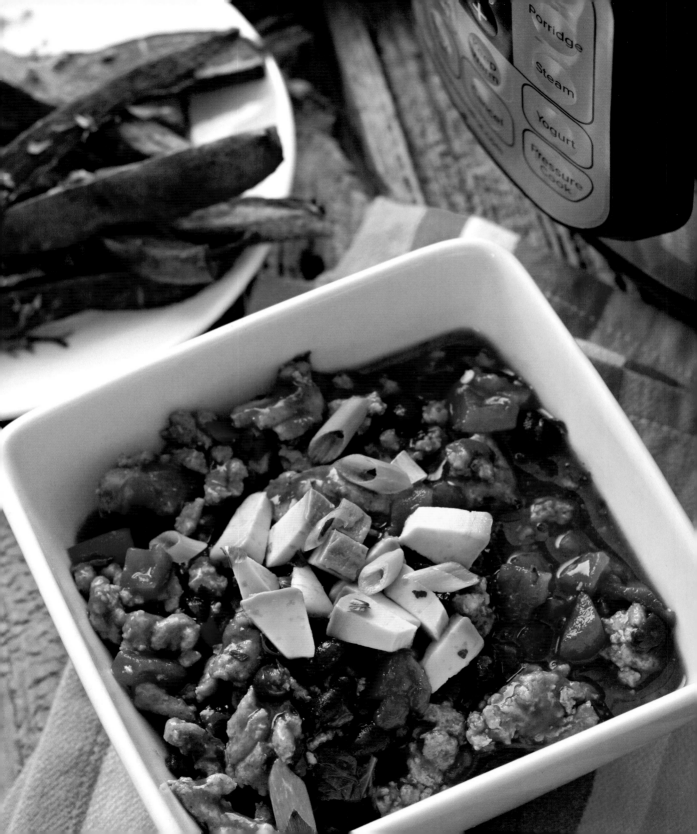

Ground Turkey Stew

Carol Eveleth, Cheyenne, WY

Makes 4–6 servings
Prep. Time: 5 minutes ⚜ Cooking Time: 25 minutes ⚜ Setting: Manual
Pressure: High ⚜ Release: Manual

I tablespoon olive oil
I onion, chopped
I pound ground turkey
½ teaspoon garlic powder
I teaspoon chili powder
¾ teaspoon cumin
2 teaspoons coriander
I teaspoon dried oregano
½ teaspoon salt
I green pepper, chopped
I red pepper, chopped
I tomato, chopped
I½ cups reduced-sodium tomato sauce
I tablespoon low-sodium soy sauce
I cup water
2 handfuls cilantro, chopped
15-ounce can reduced-salt black beans

1. Press the Sauté function on the control panel of the Instant Pot.

2. Add the olive oil to the inner pot and let it get hot. Add onion and sauté for a few minutes, or until light golden.

3. Add ground turkey. Break the ground meat using a wooden spoon to avoid formation of lumps. Sauté for a few minutes, until the pink color has faded.

4. Add garlic powder, chili powder, cumin, coriander, dried oregano, and salt. Combine well. Add green pepper, red pepper, and chopped tomato. Combine well.

5. Add tomato sauce, soy sauce, and water; combine well.

6. Close and secure the lid. Click on the Cancel key to cancel the Sauté mode. Make sure the pressure release valve on the lid is in the sealing position.

7. Click on Manual function first and then select high pressure. Click the + button and set the time to 15 minutes.

8. You can either have the steam release naturally (it will take around 20 minutes) or, after 10 minutes, turn the pressure release valve on the lid to venting and release steam. Be careful as the steam is very hot. After the pressure has released completely, open the lid.

Continued on next page . . .

9. If the stew is watery, turn on the Sauté function and let it cook for a few more minutes with the lid off.

10. Add cilantro and can of black beans, combine well, and let cook for a few minutes.

Serving suggestion:

You can serve this with whole wheat pasta—add pasta into a bowl and add reduced-fat cheddar cheese on top.

Exchange List Values	Basic Nutritional Values	
Starch 2.0	Calories 209 (Calories	Cholesterol 37 mg
Fat 0.0	from Fat 27)	Sodium 609 mg
Meat—very lean 2.0	Total Fat 3 gm	Total Carb 21 gm
Vegetable 1.5	(Saturated Fat 0.8 gm, Polyunsat Fat 0.4 gm, Monounsat Fat 1.7 gm)	Dietary Fiber 6 gm
		Sugars 8 gm
		Protein 24 gm

Green Chile Corn Chowder

Kelly Amos, Pittsboro, NC

Makes 8 servings
Prep. Time: 20 minutes ♣ Cooking Time: 7–8 hours ♣ Setting: Slow Cook

16-ounce can cream-style corn

3 potatoes, peeled and diced

2 tablespoons chopped fresh chives

4-ounce can diced green chilies, drained

2-ounce jar chopped pimentos, drained

½ cup chopped cooked ham

2 10½-ounce cans 100% fat-free lower-sodium chicken broth

Pepper to taste

Tabasco sauce to taste

1 cup fat-free milk

1. Combine all ingredients, except milk, in the inner pot of the Instant Pot.

2. Secure the lid and cook using the Slow Cook function on low 7–8 hours or until potatoes are tender.

3. When cook time is up, remove the lid and stir in the milk. Cover and let simmer another 20 minutes.

Exchange List Values

Starch 1.5

Basic Nutritional Values

Calories 124 (Calories from Fat 16)
Total Fat 2 gm
   (Saturated Fat 0.5 gm, Polyunsat Fat 0.3 gm, Monounsat Fat 0.7 gm)

Cholesterol 7 mg
Sodium 563 mg
Total Carb 21 gm
Dietary Fiber 2 gm
Sugars 7 gm
Protein 6 gm

Beef Stew

Carol Eveleth, Cheyenne, WY

Makes 6 servings
Prep. Time: 10 minutes ⚹ Cooking Time: 65 minutes ⚹ Setting: Sauté and Manual
Pressure: High ⚹ Release: Manual

2 pounds chuck steak, 1½-inch thickness

Salt to taste

Black pepper to taste

1 tablespoon Worcestershire sauce

1 tablespoon low-sodium soy sauce

3 tablespoons low-sodium tomato paste

1½ cups low-sodium chicken stock

12 white mushrooms, thinly sliced

2 small onions, thinly sliced

Olive oil, *optional*

3 cloves garlic, crushed and minced

2 celery stalks, cut into 1½-inch chunks

2 carrots, cut into 1½-inch chunks

¼ cup apple juice

2 bay leaves

¼ teaspoon dried thyme

3–4 small Yukon gold potatoes, quartered

1 tablespoon flour

½ cup frozen peas

1. Heat up your Instant Pot by pressing the Sauté button and click the adjust button to go to Sauté More function. Wait until the indicator says "hot."

2. Season one side of the chuck steak generously with salt and ground black pepper. Add olive oil into the inner pot. Be sure to coat the oil over whole bottom of the pot.

3. Carefully place the seasoned side of chuck steak in the inner pot. Generously season the other side with salt and ground black pepper. Brown for 6–8 minutes on each side without constantly flipping the steak. Remove and set aside in a large mixing bowl.

4. While the chuck steak is browning, mix together the Worcestershire sauce, soy sauce, and tomato paste with the chicken stock.

5. Add sliced mushrooms into the Instant Pot. Sauté until all moisture from the mushrooms has evaporated and the edges are slightly crisped and browned, about 6 minutes. Taste and season with salt and ground black pepper if necessary. Remove and set aside.

Exchange List Values	Basic Nutritional Values	
Starch 2.5	Calories 445 (Calories from Fat 225)	Cholesterol 103 mg
Fat 2.0		Sodium 363 mg
Meat—medium 3.0	Total Fat 25 gm (Saturated Fat 10.7 gm, Polyunsat Fat 1.2 gm, Monounsat Fat 11.7 gm)	Total Carb 23 gm
Vegetable 1.5		Dietary Fiber 4 gm
		Sugars 6 gm
		Protein 33 gm

6. Add olive oil into Instant Pot if necessary. Add onions and sauté until softened and slightly browned. Add garlic and stir for roughly 30 seconds until fragrant.

7. Add all celery and carrots and sauté until slightly browned. Season with salt and freshly ground black pepper if necessary.

8. Pour in apple juice and completely deglaze bottom of the pot by scrubbing the flavorful brown bits with a wooden spoon.

9. Add 2 bay leaves, dried thyme, quartered potatoes, and chicken stock mixture in the pot. Mix well. Close and secure lid and pressure cook on Manual at high pressure for 4 minutes. When time is up, quick release the pressure. Open the lid.

10. While the vegetables are pressure cooking, cut the chuck steak into 1-inch cubes on a large chopping board.

11. Place all chuck stew meat and the flavorful meat juice back in the large mixing bowl. Add flour in mixing bowl and mix well with the stew meat.

12. Remove half of the carrots, celery, and potatoes from pressure cooker and set aside. Place beef stew meat and all its juice in the inner pot. Partially submerge the beef stew meat in the liquid without stirring, as you don't want too much flour in the liquid at this point.

13. Close and secure the lid and pressure cook on Manual at high pressure for 32 minutes. When time is up, turn off the Instant Pot and quick release any remaining pressure.

14. On medium heat by pressing the Sauté button, break down the mushy potatoes and carrots with a wooden spoon. Stir to thicken the stew.

15. Add frozen peas, sautéed mushrooms, and the set-aside carrots, celery, and potatoes in the pot. Taste and season with salt and ground black pepper if necessary.

16. Serve with mashed potatoes, pasta, or your favorite starch. Enjoy!

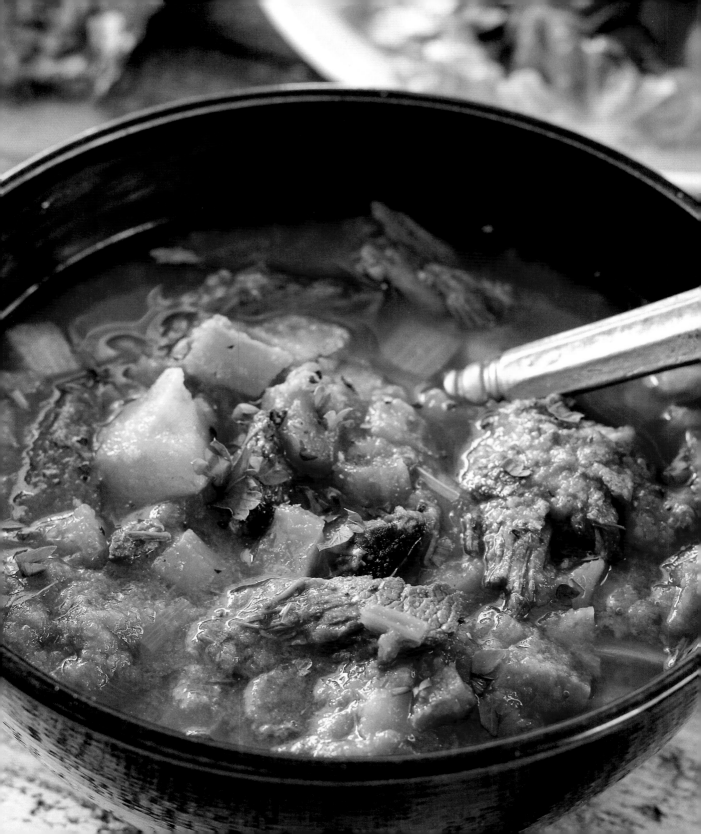

Instantly Good Beef Stew

Hope Comerford, Clinton Township, MI

Makes 6 servings

Prep. Time: 20 minutes & Cooking Time: 35 minutes & Setting: Sauté and Manual
Pressure: High & Release: Natural then Manual

3 tablespoons olive oil, *divided*

2 pounds stewing beef, cubed

2 cloves garlic, minced

1 large onion, chopped

3 ribs celery, sliced

3 large potatoes, cubed

2–3 carrots, sliced

8 ounces no-salt-added tomato sauce

10 ounces low-sodium beef broth

2 teaspoons Worcestershire sauce

¼ teaspoon pepper

1 bay leaf

1. Set the Instant Pot to the Sauté function, then add in 1 tablespoon of the oil. Add in ⅓ of the beef cubes and brown and sear all sides. Repeat this process twice more with the remaining oil and beef cubes. Set the beef aside.

2. Place the garlic, onion, and celery into the pot and sauté for a few minutes. Press Cancel.

3. Add the beef back in as well as all of the remaining ingredients.

4. Secure the lid and make sure the vent is set to sealing. Choose Manual for 35 minutes.

5. When cook time is up, let the pressure release naturally for 15 minutes, then release any remaining pressure manually.

6. Remove the lid, remove the bay leaf, then serve.

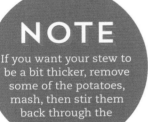

NOTE

If you want your stew to be a bit thicker, remove some of the potatoes, mash, then stir them back through the stew.

Exchange List Values

Starch 2.0

Fat 0.0

Meat—medium 4.0

Vegetable 1.0

Basic Nutritional Values

Calories 401 (Calories from Fat 180)

Total Fat 20 gm (Saturated Fat 6.2 gm, Polyunsat Fat 1.3 gm, Monounsat Fat 10.5 gm)

Cholesterol 84 mg

Sodium 157 mg

Total Carb 19 gm

Dietary Fiber 3 gm

Sugars 5 gm

Protein 35 gm

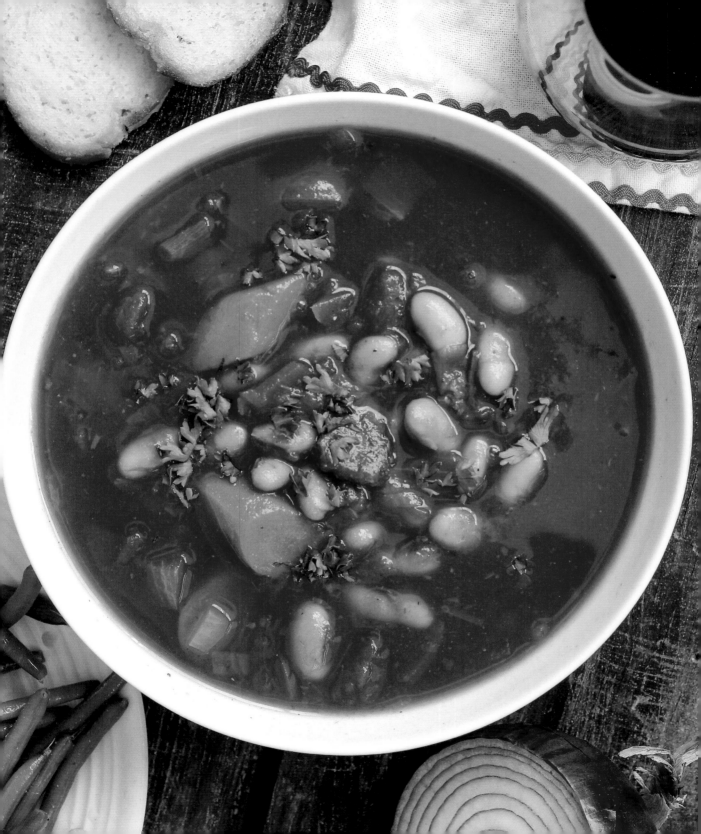

Tuscan Beef Stew

Karen Ceneviva, Seymour, CT

Makes 8 servings
Prep Time: 5–10 minutes   Cooking Time: 4–9 hours   Setting: Slow Cook

10½-ounce can tomato soup

10½-ounce can fat-free, low-sodium beef broth

½ cup water

1 teaspoon Italian seasoning

½ teaspoons garlic powder

14½-ounce can Italian diced tomatoes

¾ pound carrot chunks (1" pieces)

2 pounds stewing beef, cut into 1" cubes

2 15½-ounce cans cannellini beans, rinsed and drained

1. Mix all ingredients except beans in the inner pot of the Instant Pot.

2. Secure the lid and set the Instant Pot to the Slow Cook mode on high for 4–5 hours, or on low 8–9 hours, or until vegetables and beef are tender.

3. Remove the lid, add in the beans, and cook on Slow Cook mode once more, high for 10 more minutes.

Exchange List Values

Starch 1.0
Vegetable 1.0
Meat—lean 4.0

Basic Nutritional Values

Calories 260 (Calories from Fat 45)
Total Fat 5 gm
(Saturated Fat 2.0 gm, Polyunsat Fat 0.5 gm, Monounsat Fat 2.5 gm)

Cholesterol 60 mg
Sodium 495 mg
Total Carb 25 gm
Dietary Fiber 6 gm
Sugars 6 gm
Protein 29 gm

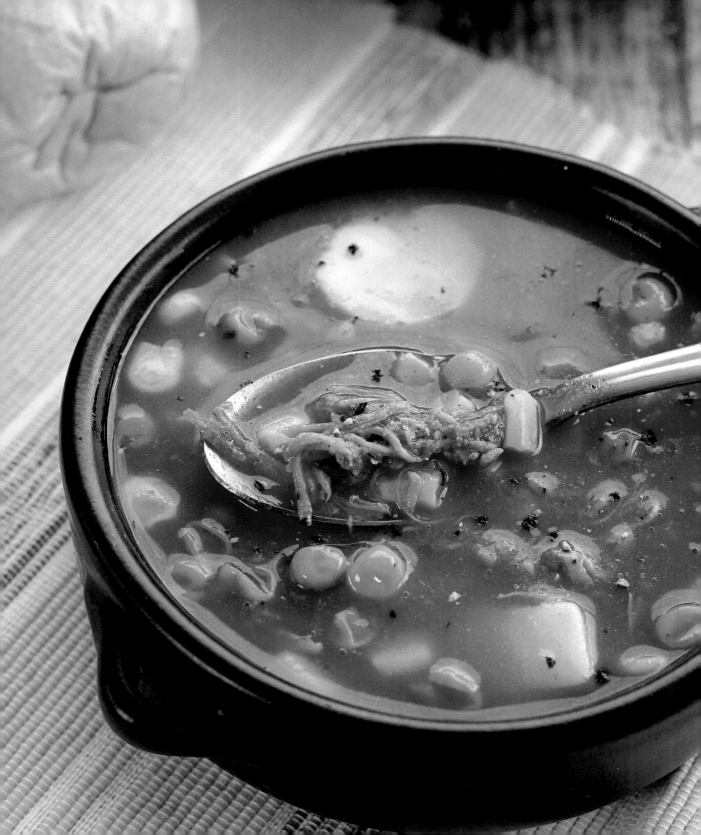

Easy Southern Brunswick Stew

Barbara Sparks, Glen Burnie, MD

Makes 12 servings
Prep. Time: 20 minutes ⚭ Cooking Time: 7–9 hours ⚭ Setting: Slow Cook

2 pounds pork butt, visible fat removed

17-ounce can white corn

1¼ cups ketchup

2 cups diced, cooked potatoes

10-ounce package frozen peas

2 10¾-ounce cans reduced-sodium
tomato soup

Hot sauce to taste, *optional*

1. Place pork in the Instant Pot and secure the lid.

2. Press the Slow Cook setting and cook on low 6–8 hours.

3. When cook time is over, remove the meat from the bone and shred, removing and discarding all visible fat.

4. Combine all the meat and remaining ingredients (except the hot sauce) in the inner pot of the Instant Pot.

5. Secure the lid once more and cook in Slow Cook mode on low for 30 minutes more. Add hot sauce if you wish.

Exchange List Values

Starch 1.0

Vegetable 2.0

Meat—lean 1.0

Fat 0.5

Basic Nutritional Values

Calories 213 (Calories from Fat 61)

Total Fat 7 gm
(Saturated Fat 2.3 gm, Polyunsat Fat 0.9 gm, Monounsat Fat 2.6 gm)

Cholesterol 34 mg

Sodium 584 mg

Total Carb 27 gm

Dietary Fiber 3 gm

Sugars 9 gm

Protein 13 gm

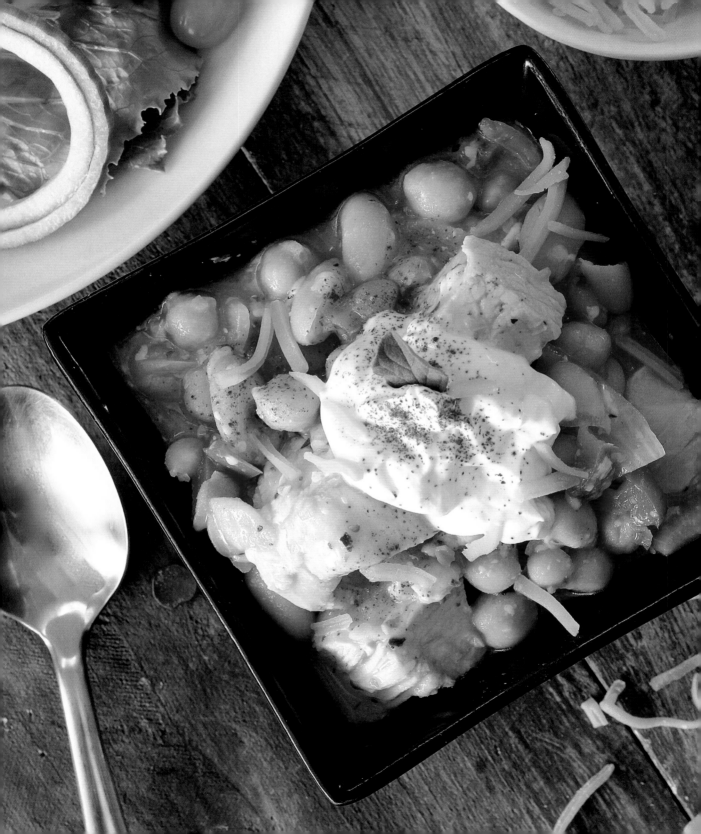

White Chicken Chili

Judy Gascho, Woodburn, OR

Makes 6 servings
Prep. Time: 20 minutes ⚜ Cooking Time: 30 minutes ⚜ Setting: Bean/Chili
Pressure: High ⚜ Release: Natural then Manual

2 tablespoons olive oil

1½–2 pounds boneless chicken breasts or thighs

1 medium onion, chopped

3 cloves garlic, minced

2 cups low-sodium chicken broth

3 15-ounce cans low-sodium great northern beans, undrained

15-ounce can low-sodium white corn, drained

4½-ounce can chopped green chilies, undrained

1 teaspoon cumin

½ teaspoon ground oregano

1 cup low-fat sour cream

1½ cups reduced-fat grated cheddar or Mexican blend cheese

1. Set Instant Pot to Sauté and allow the inner pot to get hot.

2. Add oil and chicken. Brown chicken on both sides.

3. Add onion, garlic, chicken broth, undrained beans, drained corn, undrained green chilies, cumin, and oregano.

4. Place lid on and close valve to sealing.

5. Set to Bean/Chili for 30 minutes.

6. Let pressure release naturally for 15 minutes before carefully releasing any remaining steam.

7. Remove chicken and shred.

8. Put chicken, sour cream, and cheese in the inner pot. Stir until cheese is melted.

Serving suggestion:
Can serve with chopped cilantro and additional reduced-fat cheese.

Exchange List Values

Starch 8.5
Fat 1.5
Meat—lean 3.0
Vegetable 5.0

Basic Nutritional Values

Calories 686 (Calories from Fat 63)
Total Fat 17 gm
    (Saturated Fat 4.8 gm, Polyunsat Fat 2.8 gm, Monounsat Fat 5.9 gm)

Cholesterol 131 mg
Sodium 768 mg
Total Carb 76 gm
Dietary Fiber 4 gm
Sugars 4 gm
Protein 57 gm

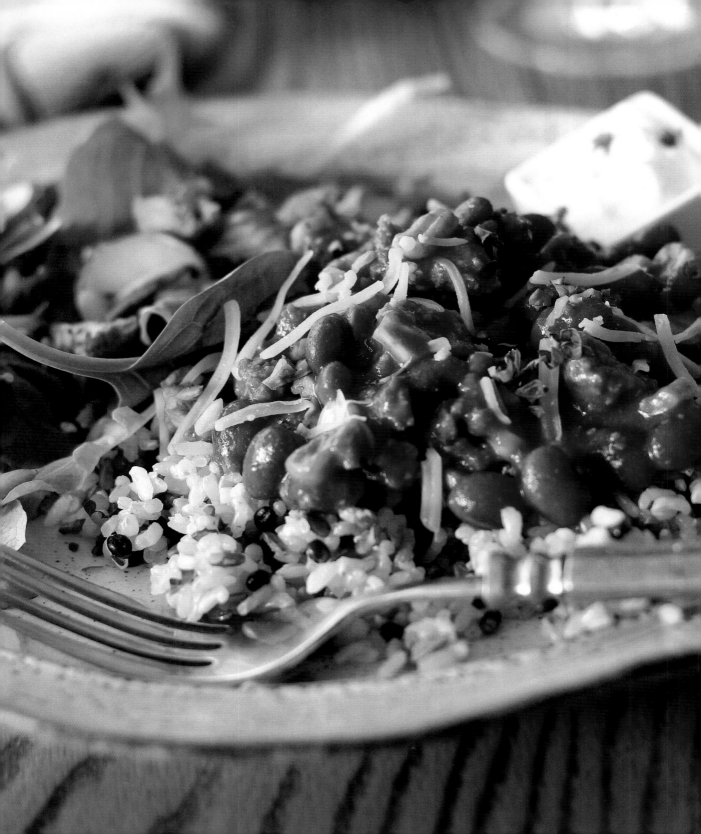

Turkey Chili

Reita F. Yoder, Carlsbad, NM

Makes 8 servings
Prep. Time: 20 minutes ⚹ Cooking Time: 5 minutes ⚹ Setting: Sauté then Manual
Pressure: High ⚹ Release: Natural then Manual

2 pounds ground turkey

1 small onion, chopped

1 garlic clove, minced

16-ounce can low-sodium pinto or kidney beans

2 cups chopped fresh tomatoes

2 cups no-salt-added tomato sauce

16-ounce can Rotel tomatoes

1-ounce package low-sodium chili seasoning

1. Turn the Instant Pot to Sauté and add a touch of olive oil or cooking spray to the inner pot. Crumble ground turkey in the inner pot and brown on the Sauté setting until cooked. Add in onions and garlic and sauté an additional 5 minutes, stirring constantly.

2. Add remaining ingredients to inner pot and mix well.

3. Secure the lid and make sure the vent is set to sealing. Cook on Manual for 5 minutes.

4. When cook time is up, let the pressure release naturally for 10 minutes, then manually release the rest.

Exchange List Values

Starch 2.0
Fat 0.0
Meat—very lean 3.5
Vegetable 1.0

Basic Nutritional Values

Calories 196 (Calories from Fat 12)
Total Fat 1.3 gm (Saturated Fat 0.5 gm, Polyunsat Fat 0.2 gm, Monounsat Fat 0.0 gm)

Cholesterol 55 mg
Sodium 380 mg
Total Carb 15 gm
Dietary Fiber 3 gm
Sugars 7 gm
Protein 31 gm

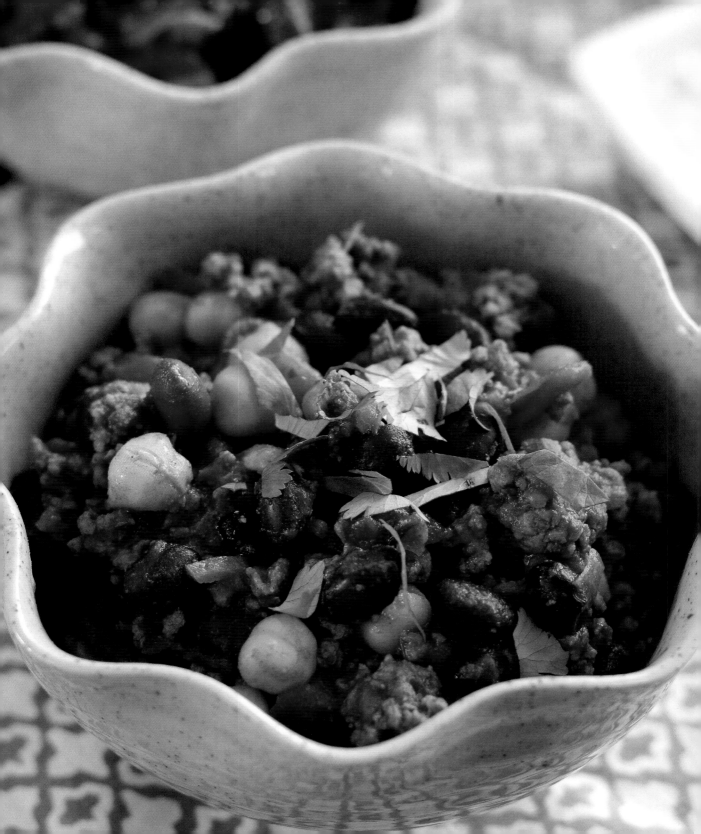

Three-Bean Chili

Chris Kaczynski, Schenectady, NY

Makes 6 servings
Prep. Time: 30 minutes ⚘ *Cooking Time: 15 minutes* ⚘ *Setting: Sauté and Manual*
Pressure: High ⚘ *Release: Natural then Manual*

1 pound extra-lean ground beef

1 medium onion, diced

1 cup medium salsa

1 package low-sodium dry chili seasoning

1 16-ounce can low-sodium red kidney beans, drained

1 16-ounce can low-sodium black beans, drained

1 16-ounce can low-sodium white kidney, or garbanzo, beans drained

14-ounce can low-sodium crushed tomatoes

14-ounce can low-sodium diced tomatoes

5 drops liquid stevia

1. Turn the Instant Pot to Sauté and add a touch of olive oil or cooking spray to the inner pot. Brown the beef and onion. Press Cancel when done.

2. Stir in the remaining ingredients.

3. Secure the lid and make sure vent is set to sealing. Press Manual and set for 15 minutes.

4. When cooking time is done, let the pressure release naturally for 10 minutes and then manually release the rest.

Exchange List Values

Starch 2.5
Fat 1.0
Meat—lean 1.5
Vegetable 1.5

Basic Nutritional Values

Calories 245 (Calories from Fat 72)
Total Fat 8 gm
(Saturated Fat 3.0 gm, Polyunsat Fat 0.6 gm, Monounsat Fat 3.2 gm)
Cholesterol 49 mg
Sodium 589 mg
Total Carb 22 gm
Dietary Fiber 6 gm
Sugars 6 gm
Protein 21 gm

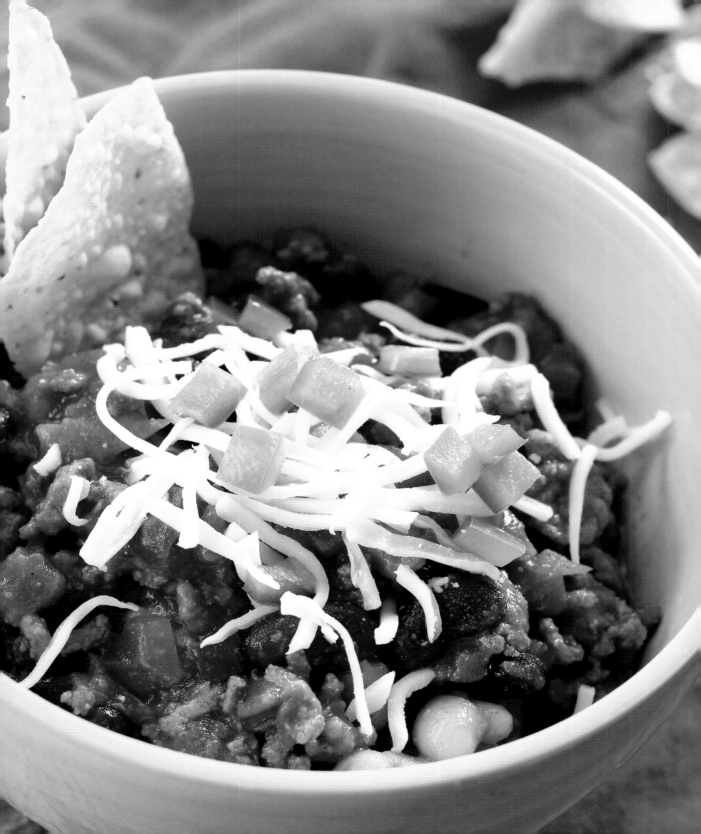

Favorite Chili

Carol Eveleth, Cheyenne, WY

Makes 4–6 servings
Prep. Time: 10 minutes ⚜ Cooking Time: 35 minutes ⚜ Setting: Manual
Pressure: High ⚜ Release: Natural

1 pound extra-lean ground beef
1 teaspoon salt
½ teaspoons black pepper
1 tablespoon olive oil
1 small onion, chopped
2 cloves garlic, minced
1 green pepper, chopped
2 tablespoons chili powder
½ teaspoons cumin
1 cup water
16-ounce can chili beans
15-ounce can low-sodium crushed tomatoes

1. Press Sauté button and adjust once to Sauté More function. Wait until indicator says "hot."

2. Season the ground beef with salt and black pepper.

3. Add the olive oil into the inner pot. Coat the whole bottom of the pot with the oil.

4. Add ground beef into the inner pot. The ground beef will start to release moisture. Allow the ground beef to brown and crisp slightly, stirring occasionally to break it up. Taste and adjust the seasoning with more salt and ground black pepper.

5. Add diced onion, minced garlic, chopped pepper, chili powder, and cumin. Sauté for about 5 minutes, until the spices start to release their fragrance. Stir frequently.

6. Add water and 1 can of chili beans, not drained. Mix well. Pour in 1 can of crushed tomatoes.

7. Close and secure lid, making sure vent is set to sealing, and pressure cook on Manual at high pressure for 10 minutes.

8. Let the pressure release naturally when cooking time is up. Open the lid carefully.

Serving suggestion:
Garnish chili with low-fat sour cream, reduced-fat shredded cheese, jalepeño slices, or chopped onions.

Exchange List Values	Basic Nutritional Values	
Starch 1.0	Calories 213 (Calories from Fat 90)	Cholesterol 49 mg
Fat 0.0		Sodium 385 mg
Meat—medium 2.0	Total Fat 10 gm	Total Carb 11 gm
Vegetable 1.0	(Saturated Fat 3.4 gm, Polyunsat Fat 0.6 gm, Monounsat Fat 4.9 gm)	Dietary Fiber 4 gm
		Sugars 4 gm
		Protein 18 gm

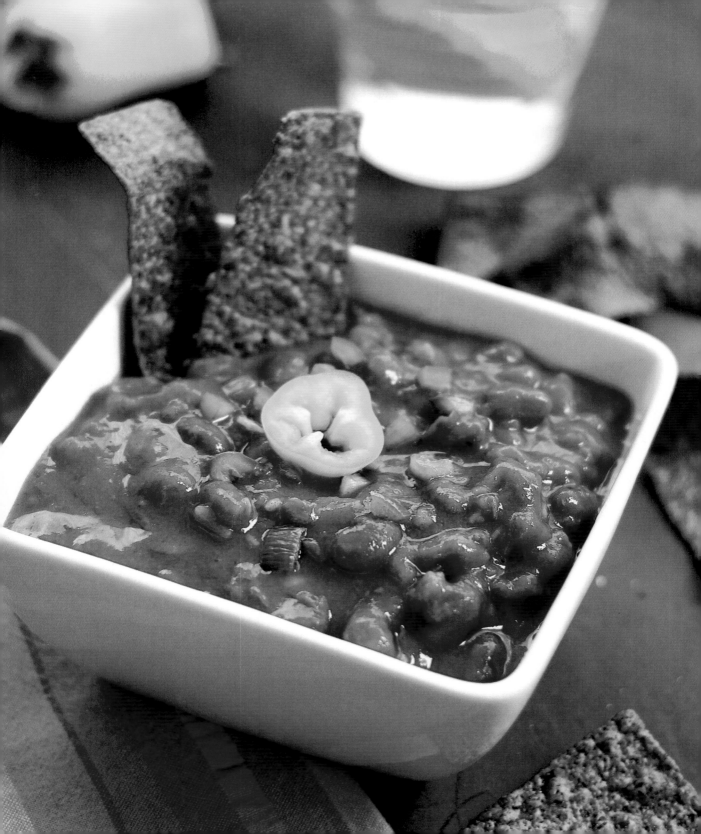

Vegetarian Chili

Connie Johnson, Loudon, NH

Makes 6 servings
Prep. Time: 25 minutes ⚹ Cooking Time: 10 minutes ⚹ Setting: Manual
Pressure: High ⚹ Release: Natural then Manual

2 teaspoons olive oil

3 garlic cloves, minced

2 onions, chopped

1 green bell pepper, chopped

1 cup textured vegetable protein (T.V.P.)

1-pound can beans of your choice, drained

1 jalapeño pepper, seeds removed, chopped

28-ounce can diced Italian tomatoes

1 bay leaf

1 tablespoon dried oregano

½ teaspoons salt

¼ teaspoons pepper

1. Set the Instant Pot to the Sauté function. As it's heating, add the olive oil, garlic, onions, and bell pepper. Stir constantly for about 5 minutes as it all cooks. Press Cancel.

2. Place all of the remaining ingredients into the inner pot of the Instant pot and stir.

3. Secure the lid and make sure vent is set to sealing. Cook on Manual mode for 10 minutes.

4. When cook time is up, let the steam release naturally for 5 minutes and then manually release the rest.

Exchange List Values

Starch 4.0

Fat 0.5

Vegetable 2.5

Basic Nutritional Values

Calories 242 (Calories from Fat 18)

Total Fat 2 gm (Saturated Fat 0.4 gm, Polyunsat Fat 0.4 gm, Monounsat Fat 1.2 gm)

Cholesterol 0 mg

Sodium 489 mg

Total Carb 36 gm

Dietary Fiber 12 gm

Sugars 9 gm

Protein 17 gm

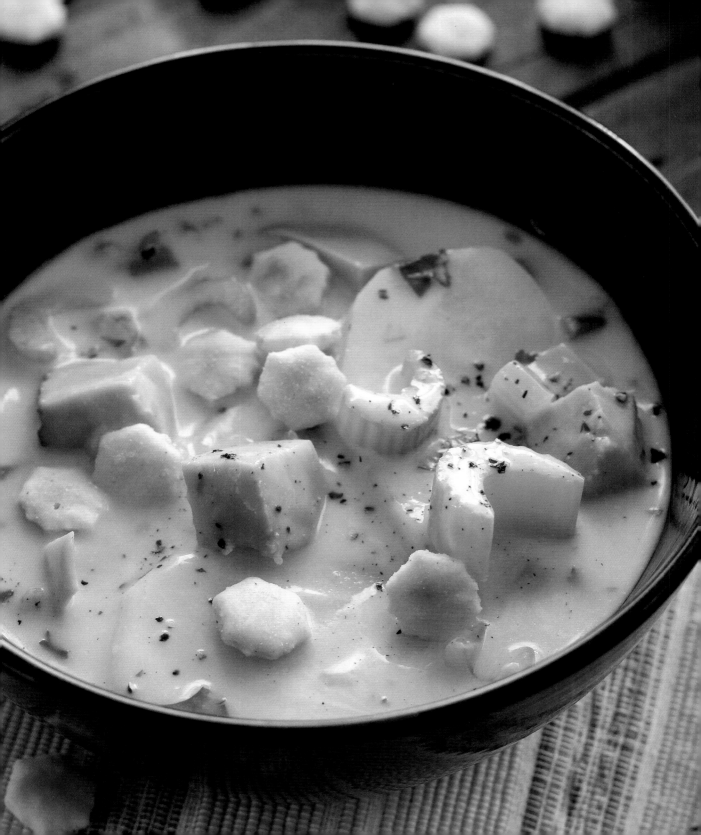

Ham and Potato Chowder

Penny Blosser, Beavercreek, OH

Makes 5 servings
Prep. Time: 25 minutes ⚭ Cooking Time: 8 hours ⚭ Setting: Slow Cook

5-ounce package scalloped potatoes

Sauce mix from potato package

1 cup extra-lean, reduced-sodium, cooked ham, cut into narrow strips

4 teaspoons sodium-free bouillon powder

4 cups water

1 cup chopped celery

⅓ cup chopped onions

Pepper to taste

2 cups fat-free half-and-half

⅓ cup flour

1. Combine potatoes, sauce mix, ham, bouillon powder, water, celery, onions, and pepper in the inner pot of the Instant Pot.

2. Secure the lid and cook using the Slow Cook function on low for 7 hours.

3. Combine half-and-half and flour. Remove the lid and gradually add to the inner pot, blending well.

4. Secure the lid once more and cook on the low Slow Cook function for up to 1 hour more, stirring occasionally until thickened.

Exchange List Values

Starch 1.5
Carbohydrate 1.0
Meat—lean 1.0

Basic Nutritional Values

Calories 241 (Calories from Fat 29)
Total Fat 3 gm
(Saturated Fat 1.2 gm, Polyunsat Fat 0.7 gm, Monounsat Fat 0.2 gm)

Cholesterol 21 mg
Sodium 836 mg
Total Carb 41 gm
Dietary Fiber 3 gm
Sugars 8 gm
Protein 11 gm

Main Dishes

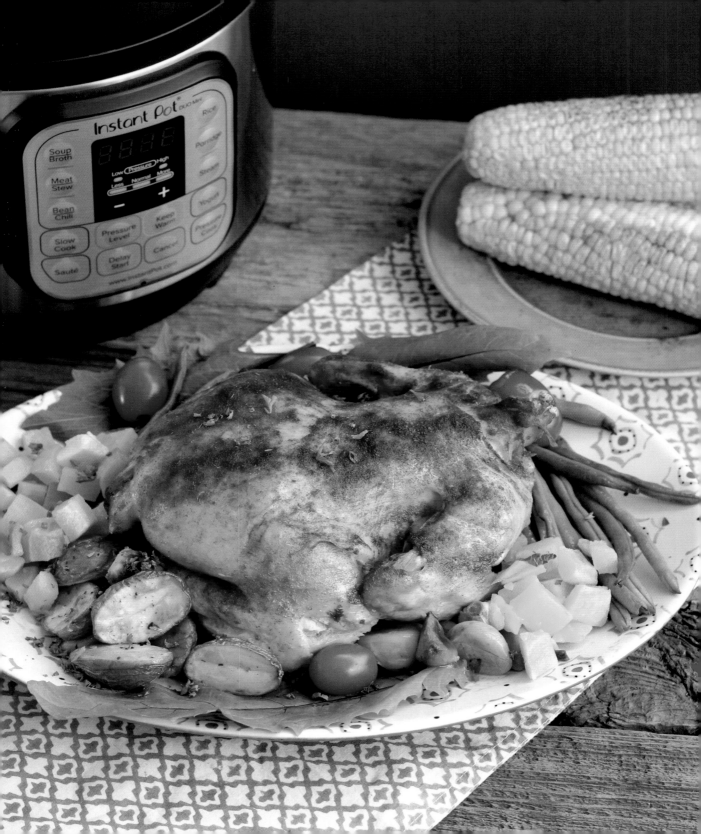

Garlic Galore Rotisserie Chicken

Hope Comerford, Clinton Township, MI

Makes 4 servings

Prep. Time: 5 minutes ⁂ *Cooking Time: 33 minutes* ⁂ *Setting: Sauté and Manual*
Pressure: High ⁂ *Release: Natural then Manual*

3-pound whole chicken
2 tablespoons olive oil, *divided*
Salt to taste
Pepper to taste
20–30 cloves fresh garlic, peeled and left whole
1 cup low-sodium chicken stock, broth, or water
2 tablespoons garlic powder
2 teaspoons onion powder
½ teaspoon basil
½ teaspoon cumin
½ teaspoon chili powder

1. Rub chicken with one tablespoon of the olive oil and sprinkle with salt and pepper.

2. Place the garlic cloves inside the chicken. Use butcher's twine to secure the legs.

3. Press the Sauté button on the Instant Pot, then add the rest of the olive oil to the inner pot.

4. When the pot is hot, place the chicken inside. You are just trying to sear it, so leave it for about 4 minutes on each side.

5. Remove the chicken and set aside. Place the trivet at the bottom of the inner pot and pour in the chicken stock.

6. Mix together the remaining seasonings and rub them all over the entire chicken.

7. Place the chicken back inside the inner pot, breast-side up, on top of the trivet and secure the lid to the sealing position.

8. Press the Manual button and use the +/- to set it for 25 minutes.

9. When the timer beeps, allow the pressure to release naturally for 15 minutes. If the lid will not open at this point, quick release the remaining pressure and remove the chicken.

10. Let the chicken rest for 5–10 minutes before serving.

Exchange List Values

Meat—medium 4.0
Fat 0.5

Basic Nutritional Values

Calories 333 (Calories from Fat 1)
Total Fat 23 gm (Saturated Fat 5.3 gm, Polyunsat Fat 3.7 gm, Monounsat Fat 12 gm)
Cholesterol 113 mg
Sodium 110 mg
Total Carb 9 gm
Dietary Fiber 1 gm
Sugars 0 gm
Protein 24 gm

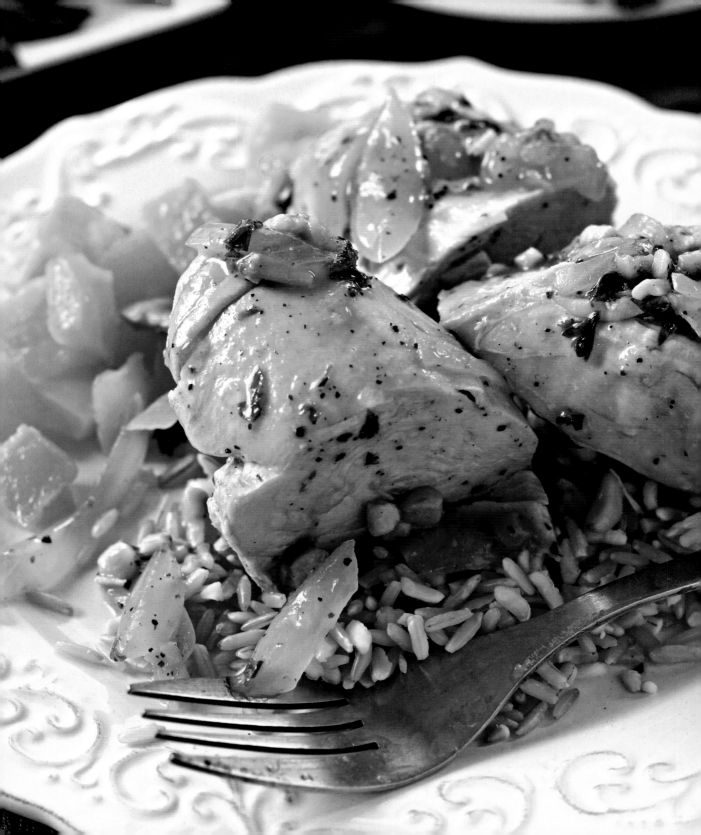

Buttery Lemon Chicken

Judy Gascho, Woodburn, OR

Makes 4 servings
Prep. Time: 15 minutes ⚹ Cooking Time: 7 minutes ⚹ Setting: Poultry
Pressure: High ⚹ Release: Natural

2 tablespoons margarine

1 medium onion, chopped

4 cloves garlic, minced

½ teaspoon paprika

½ teaspoon pepper

1 teaspoon dried parsley, or 1 tablespoon chopped fresh parsley

2 pounds boneless chicken breasts or thighs

½ cup low-sodium chicken broth

⅓ cup lemon juice

1 teaspoon salt

1–2 tablespoons cornstarch

1 tablespoon water

1. Set the Instant Pot to Sauté. When it is hot, add margarine to the inner pot and melt.

2. Add the onion, garlic, paprika, pepper, and parsley to melted margarine and sauté until onion starts to soften. Push onion to side of pot.

3. With the Instant Pot still at Sauté, add the chicken and sear on each side 3–5 minutes.

4. Mix broth, lemon juice, and salt together. Pour over chicken and stir to mix together.

5. Put on lid and set Instant Pot, move vent to sealing, and press Poultry. Set cook time for 7 minutes. Let depressurize naturally.

6. Remove chicken, leaving sauce in pot. Mix cornstarch in water and add to sauce. (Can start with 1 tablespoon cornstarch, and use second one if sauce isn't thick enough.)

Serving suggestion:
Serve chicken and sauce over noodles or rice.

Exchange List Values

Meat—lean 7.0
Fat 0.0

Basic Nutritional Values

Calories 350 (Calories from Fat 108)
Total Fat 12 gm (Saturated Fat 4.3 gm, Polyunsat Fat 2.7 gm, Monounsat Fat 4.3 gm)

Cholesterol 165 mg
Sodium 658 mg
Total Carb 6 gm
Dietary Fiber 0 gm
Sugars 1 gm
Protein 52 gm

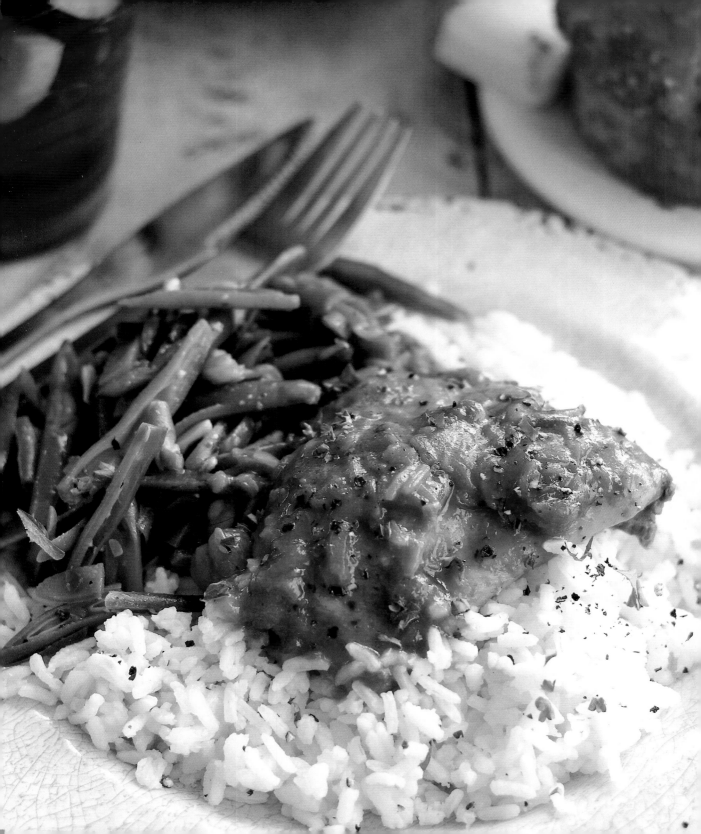

Chicken in Wine

Mary Seielstad, Sparks, NV

Makes 6 servings
Prep. Time: 10 minutes ⚬ Cooking Time: 12 minutes ⚬ Setting: Manual
Pressure: High ⚬ Release: Natural then Manual

2 pounds chicken breasts, trimmed of skin and fat

10¾-ounce can 98% fat-free, reduced-sodium cream of mushroom soup

10¾-ounce can French onion soup

1 cup dry white wine or chicken broth

1. Place the chicken into the Instant Pot.

2. Combine soups and wine. Pour over chicken.

3. Secure the lid and make sure vent is set to sealing. Cook on Manual mode for 12 minutes.

4. When cook time is up, let the pressure release naturally for 5 minutes and then release the rest manually.

Exchange List Values

Carbohydrate 0.5
Meat—very lean 5.0

Basic Nutritional Values

Calories 225 (Calories from Fat 47)
Total Fat 5 gm (Saturated Fat 1.4 gm, Polyunsat Fat 1.2 gm, Monounsat Fat 1.6 gm)

Cholesterol 91 mg
Sodium 645 mg
Total Carb 7 gm
Dietary Fiber 1 gm
Sugars 3 gm
Protein 35 gm

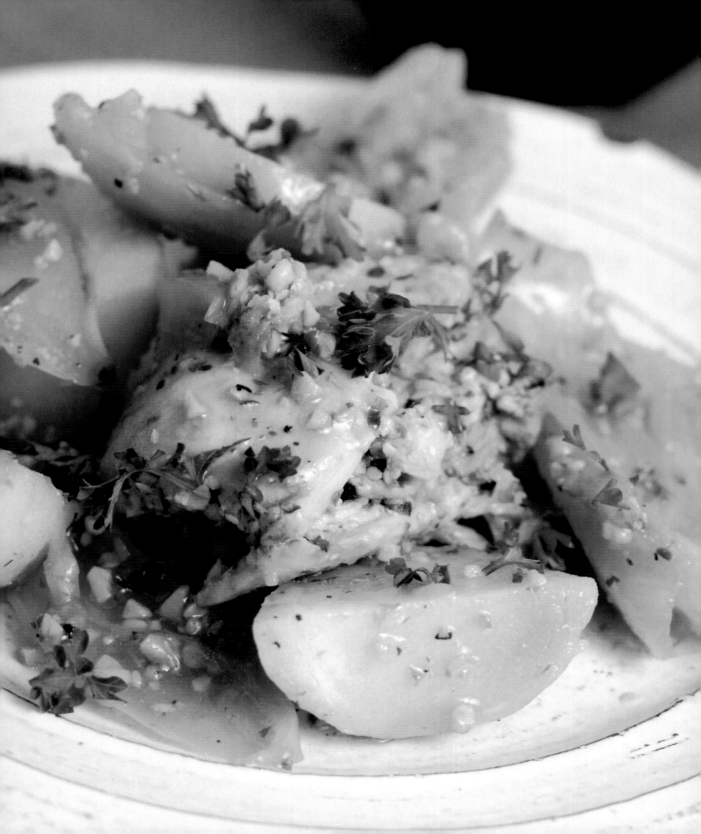

Greek Chicken

Judy Govotsos, Monrovia, MD

Makes 6 servings
Prep. Time: 25 minutes ⚹ Cooking Time: 20 minutes ⚹ Setting: Manual
Pressure: High ⚹ Release: Natural then Manual

4 potatoes, unpeeled, quartered

2 pounds chicken pieces, trimmed of skin and fat

2 large onions, quartered

1 whole bulb garlic, cloves minced

3 teaspoons dried oregano

¾ teaspoons salt

½ teaspoons pepper

1 tablespoon olive oil

1 cup water

1. Place potatoes, chicken, onions, and garlic into the inner pot of the Instant Pot, then sprinkle with seasonings. Top with oil and water.

2. Secure the lid and make sure vent is set to sealing. Cook on Manual mode for 20 minutes.

3. When cook time is over, let the pressure release naturally for 5 minutes, then release the rest manually.

Exchange List Values

Starch 1.5
Vegetable 2.0
Meat—lean 2.0

Basic Nutritional Values

Calories 278 (Calories from Fat 56)
Total Fat 6 gm
(Saturated Fat 1.3 gm, Polyunsat Fat 1.1 gm, Monounsat Fat 3.0 gm)

Cholesterol 65 mg
Sodium 358 mg
Total Carb 29 gm
Dietary Fiber 4 gm
Sugars 9 gm
Protein 27 gm

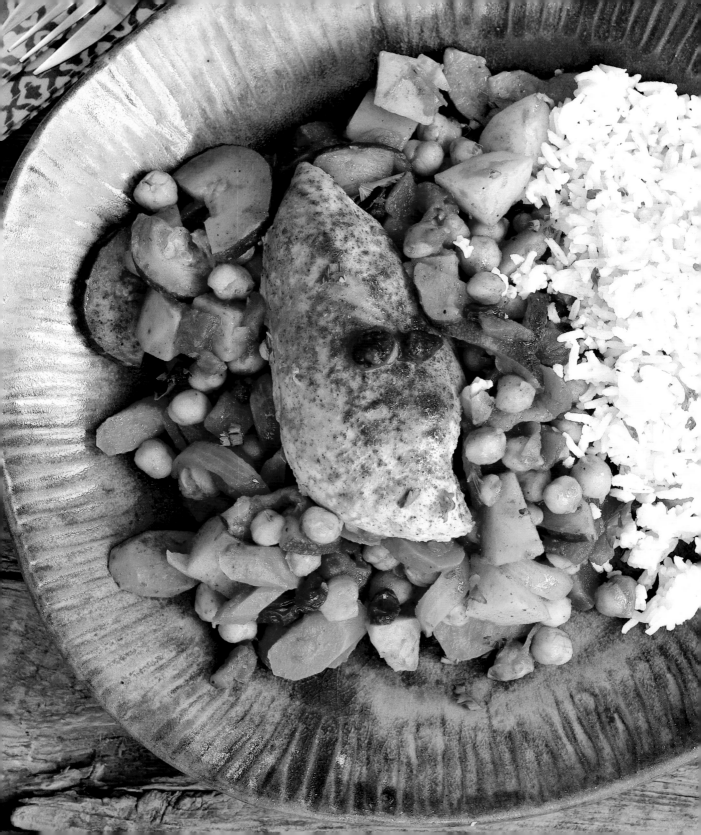

Chicken Casablanca

Joyce Kaut, Rochester, NY

Makes 8 servings
Prep. Time: 20 minutes ⚹ Cooking Time: 12 minutes ⚹ Setting: Sauté and Manual
Pressure: High ⚹ Release: Natural then Manual

2 large onions, sliced

1 teaspoon ground ginger

3 garlic cloves, minced

2 tablespoons canola oil, *divided*

3 pounds skinless chicken pieces

3 large carrots, diced

2 large potatoes, unpeeled, diced

½ teaspoon ground cumin

½ teaspoon salt

½ teaspoon pepper

¼ teaspoon cinnamon

2 tablespoons raisins

14½-ounce can chopped tomatoes

3 small zucchini, sliced

15-ounce can garbanzo beans, drained

2 tablespoons chopped parsley

1. Using the Sauté function of the Instant Pot, cook the onions, ginger, and garlic in 1 tablespoon of the oil for 5 minutes, stirring constantly. Remove onions, ginger, and garlic from pot and set aside.

2. Brown the chicken pieces with the remaining oil, then add the cooked onions, ginger and garlic back in as well as all of the remaining ingredients, except the parsley.

3. Secure the lid and make sure vent is in the sealing position. Cook on Manual mode for 12 minutes.

4. When cook time is up, let the pressure release naturally for 5 minutes and then release the rest of the pressure manually.

Exchange List Values

Starch 2.0
Vegetable 2.0
Meat—lean 3.0
Fat 0.5

Basic Nutritional Values

Calories 395 (Calories from Fat 93)
Total Fat 10 gm (Saturated Fat 1.9 gm, Polyunsat Fat 2.9 gm, Monounsat Fat 4.3 gm)

Cholesterol 87 mg
Sodium 390 mg
Total Carb 40 gm
Dietary Fiber 8 gm
Sugars 12 gm
Protein 36 gm

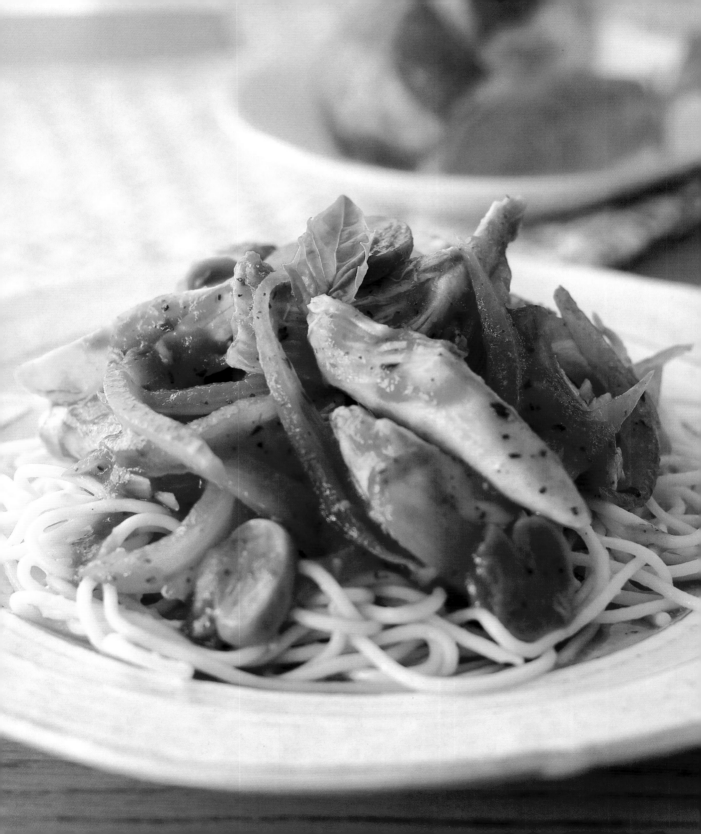

Ann's Chicken Cacciatore

Ann Driscoll, Albuquerque, NM

Makes 8 servings
Prep. Time: 25 minutes ⚭ Cooking Time: 3–9 hours ⚭ Setting: Slow Cook

1 large onion, thinly sliced

3 pound chicken, cut up, skin removed, trimmed of fat

2 6-ounce cans tomato paste

4-ounce can sliced mushrooms, drained

1 teaspoon salt

¼ cup dry white wine

¼ teaspoons pepper

1–2 garlic cloves, minced

1–2 teaspoons dried oregano

½ teaspoon dried basil

½ teaspoon celery seed, *optional*

1 bay leaf

1. In the inner pot of the Instant Pot, place the onion and chicken.

2. Combine remaining ingredients and pour over the chicken.

3. Secure the lid and make sure vent is at sealing. Cook on Slow Cook mode, low 7–9 hours, or high 3–4 hours.

Exchange List Values

Vegetable 3.0
Meat—lean 2.0

Basic Nutritional Values

Calories 161 (Calories from Fat 40)
Total Fat 4 gm (Saturated Fat 1.1 gm, Polyunsat Fat 1.1 gm, Monounsat Fat 1.5 gm)
Cholesterol 49 mg
Sodium 405 mg
Total Carb 12 gm
Dietary Fiber 3 gm
Sugars 3 gm
Protein 19 gm

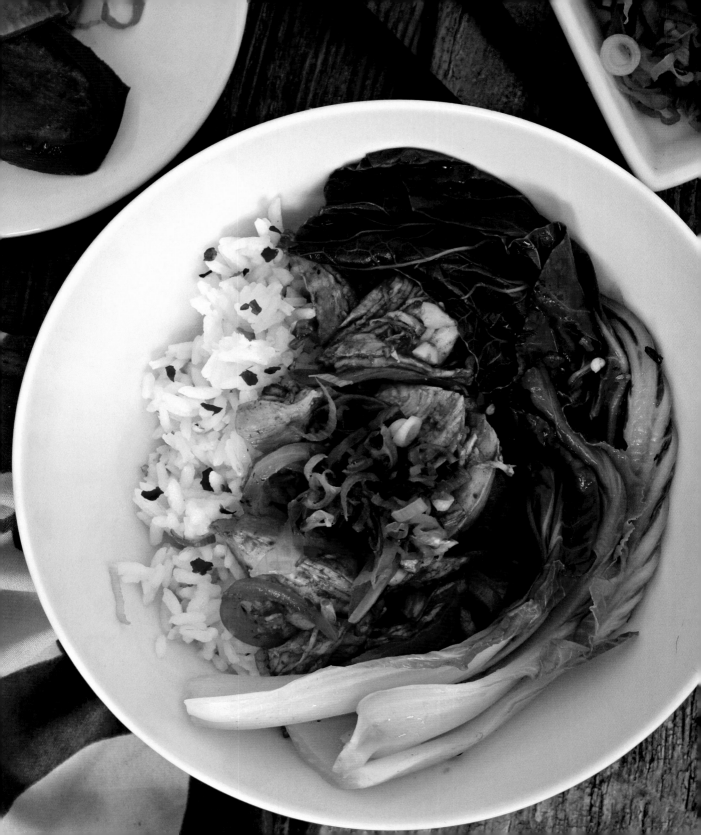

Chicken with Spiced Sesame Sauce

Colleen Heatwole, Burton, MI

Makes 4–6 servings
Prep. Time: 20 minutes ⚸ Cooking Time: 8 minutes ⚸ Setting: Manual
Pressure: High ⚸ Release: Manual

2 tablespoons tahini (sesame sauce)

¼ cup water

1 tablespoon low-sodium soy sauce

¼ cup chopped onion

1 teaspoon red wine vinegar

2 teaspoons minced garlic

1 teaspoon shredded ginger root
(Microplane works best)

2 pounds chicken breast, chopped into
8 portions

1. Place first seven ingredients in bottom of the inner pot of the Instant Pot.

2. Add coarsely chopped chicken on top.

3. Secure the lid and make sure vent is at sealing. Set for 8 minutes using Manual setting. When cook time is up, let the pressure release naturally for 10 minutes, then perform a quick release.

4. Remove ingredients and shred chicken with fork. Combine with other ingredients in pot for a tasty sandwich filling or sauce.

Exchange List Values

Meat—lean 5.0
Fat 0.0

Basic Nutritional Values

Calories 215 (Calories from Fat 63)
Total Fat 7 gm
(Saturated Fat 1.2 gm, Polyunsat Fat 1.8 gm, Monounsat Fat 2.0 gm)

Cholesterol 110 mg
Sodium 178 mg
Total Carb 2 gm
Dietary Fiber 0 gm
Sugars 0 gm
Protein 35 gm

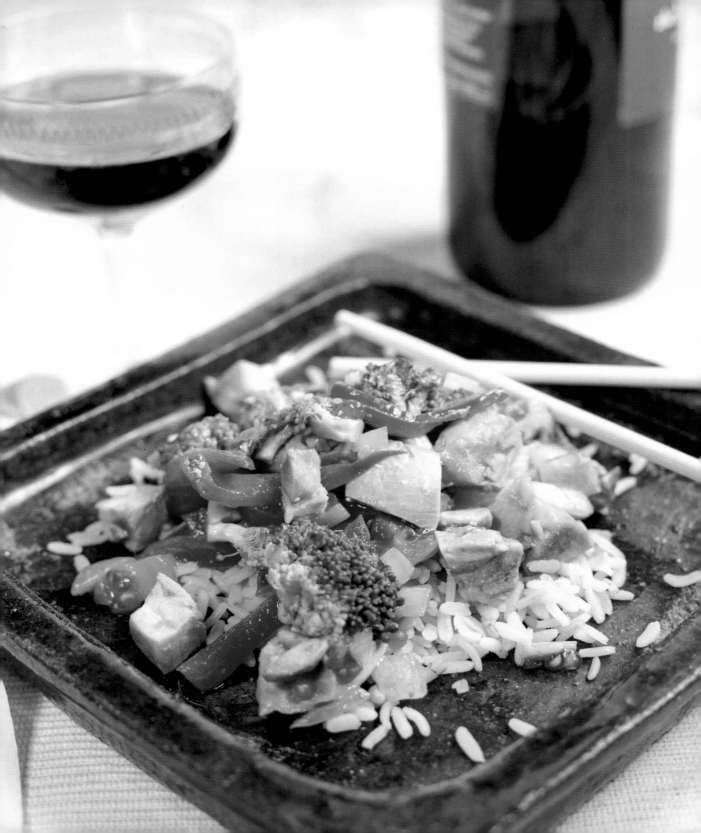

Szechuan-Style Chicken and Broccoli

Jane Meiser, Harrisonburg, VA

Makes 4 servings
Prep. Time: 20 minutes ⚭ Cooking Time: 12 minutes ⚭ Setting: Sauté and Manual
Pressure: High ⚭ Release: Natural then Manual

1 tablespoon canola oil

2 whole boneless, skinless chicken breasts, cut into 1" cubes

2 cups broccoli florets

1 medium red bell pepper, sliced

½ cup picante sauce

½ cup low-sodium chicken stock

2 tablespoons light soy sauce

½ teaspoon sugar

2 teaspoons quick-cooking tapioca

1 medium onion, chopped

2 garlic cloves, minced

½ teaspoon ground ginger

1. Set the Instant Pot to Sauté and add the oil and chicken. Sauté until lightly browned. Press Cancel.

2. Add in the broccoli and bell pepper. In a small bowl, mix together the remaining ingredients, then pour over the contents of the Instant Pot and stir.

3. Secure the lid and make sure vent is at sealing. Cook in Manual mode for 12 minutes.

4. When cooking time is over, let the pressure release naturally for 5 minutes, then release the rest manually.

Exchange List Values

Meat—lean 4.0
Fat 0.0

Basic Nutritional Values

Calories 217 (Calories from Fat 63)
Total Fat 7 gm
  (Saturated Fat 1.0 gm, Polyunsat Fat 1.5 gm, Monounsat Fat 2.9 gm)

Cholesterol 83 mg
Sodium 425 mg
Total Carb 11 gm
Dietary Fiber 2 gm
Sugars 5 gm
Protein 27 gm

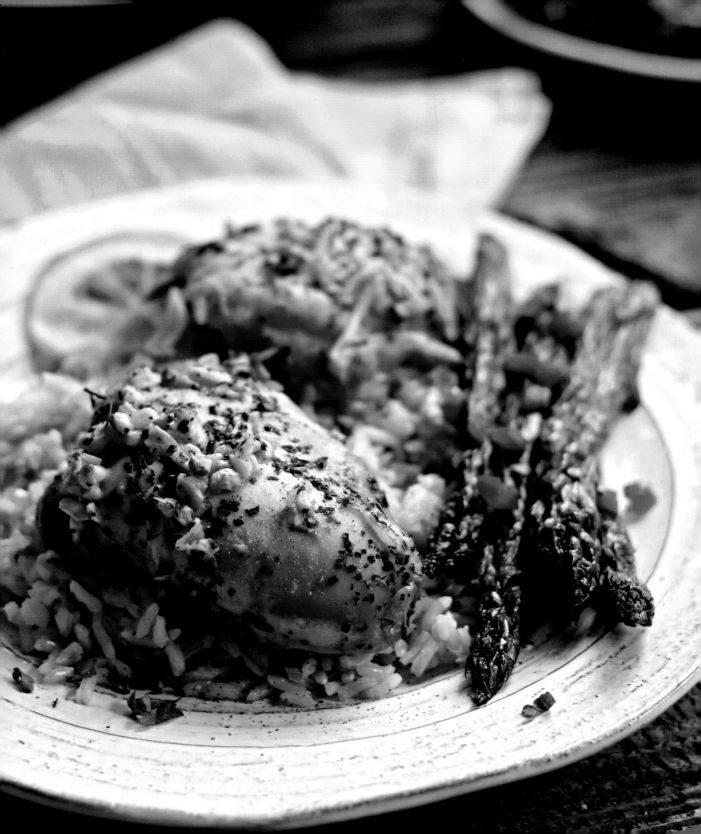

Lemony Chicken Thighs

Maria Shevlin, Sicklerville, NJ

Makes 3–5 servings
Prep. Time: 15 minutes ⚜ Cooking Time: 15 minutes ⚜ Setting: Poultry
Pressure: High ⚜ Release: Natural then Manual

1 cup low-sodium chicken bone broth

5 frozen bone-in chicken thighs

1 small onion, diced

5–6 cloves garlic, diced

Juice of 1 lemon

2 tablespoons margarine, melted

½ teaspoon salt

¼ teaspoon black pepper

1 teaspoon True Lemon Lemon Pepper seasoning

1 teaspoon parsley flakes

¼ teaspoon oregano

Rind of 1 lemon

1. Add the chicken bone broth into the inner pot of the Instant Pot.

2. Add the chicken thighs.

3. Add the onion and garlic.

4. Pour the fresh lemon juice in with the melted margarine.

5. Add the seasonings.

6. Lock the lid, make sure the vent is at sealing, then press the Poultry button. Set to 15 minutes.

7. When cook time is up, let the pressure naturally release for 3–5 minutes, then manually release the rest.

8. You can place these under the broiler for 2–3 minutes to brown.

9. Plate up and pour some of the sauce over top with fresh grated lemon rind.

Exchange List Values

Meat—medium 4.0
Fat 1.0

Basic Nutritional Values

Calories 329 (Calories from Fat 216)
Total Fat 24 gm (Saturated Fat 23.8 gm, Polyunsat Fat 5.1 gm, Monounsat Fat 11.1 gm)

Cholesterol 142 mg
Sodium 407 mg
Total Carb 3 gm
Dietary Fiber 0 gm
Sugars 1 gm
Protein 26 gm

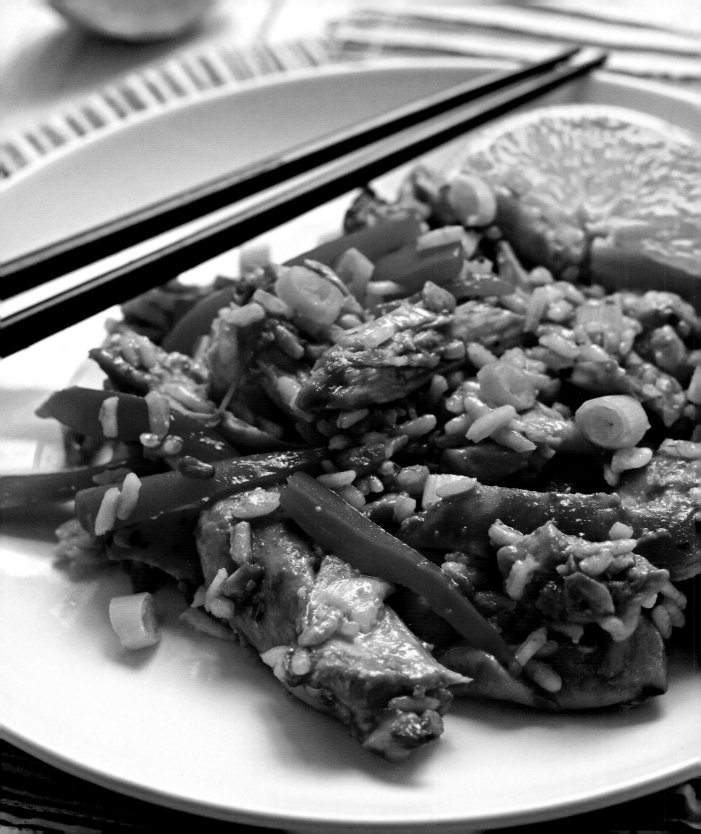

Orange Chicken Thighs with Bell Peppers

Maria Shevlin, Sicklerville, NJ

Makes 4–6 servings

Prep. Time: 15–20 minutes 🔹 Cooking Time: 7 minutes 🔹 Setting: Sauté and Manual
Pressure: High 🔹 Release: Manual

6 boneless skinless chicken thighs, cut into bite-sized pieces

2 packets crystallized True Orange flavoring

½ teaspoon True Orange Orange Ginger seasoning

½ teaspoon coconut aminos

¼ teaspoon Worcestershire sauce

Olive oil or cooking spray

2 cups bell pepper strips, any color combination (I used red)

1 onion, chopped

1 tablespoon green onion, chopped fine

3 cloves garlic, minced or chopped

½ teaspoon pink salt

½ teaspoon black pepper

1 teaspoon garlic powder

1 teaspoon ground ginger

¼–½ teaspoon red pepper flakes

2 tablespoons tomato paste

½ cup chicken bone broth or water

1 tablespoon brown sugar substitute (I use Sukrin Gold)

½ cup Seville orange spread (I use Crofter's brand)

1. Combine the chicken with the 2 packets of crystallized orange flavor, the orange ginger seasoning, the coconut aminos, and the Worcestershire sauce. Set aside.

2. Turn the Instant Pot to Sauté and add a touch of olive oil or cooking spray to the inner pot. Add in the orange ginger marinated chicken thighs.

3. Sauté until lightly browned. Add in the peppers, onion, green onion, garlic, and seasonings. Mix well.

4. Add the remaining ingredients; mix to combine.

5. Lock the lid, set the vent to sealing, set to 7 minutes.

6. Let the pressure release naturally for 2 minutes, then manually release the rest when cook time is up.

Exchange List Values

Meat—lean 2.0
Fat 0.0

Basic Nutritional Values

Calories 120 (Calories from Fat 18)
Total Fat 2 gm
   (Saturated Fat 0.6 gm, Polyunsat Fat 0.5 gm, Monounsat Fat 0.7 gm)

Cholesterol 49 mg
Sodium 315 mg
Total Carb 8 gm
Dietary Fiber 1.6 gm
Sugars 10 gm
Protein 12 gm

Serving suggestion:

Serve with your choice of pasta or rice and top with additional green onion and/or sesame seeds as well.

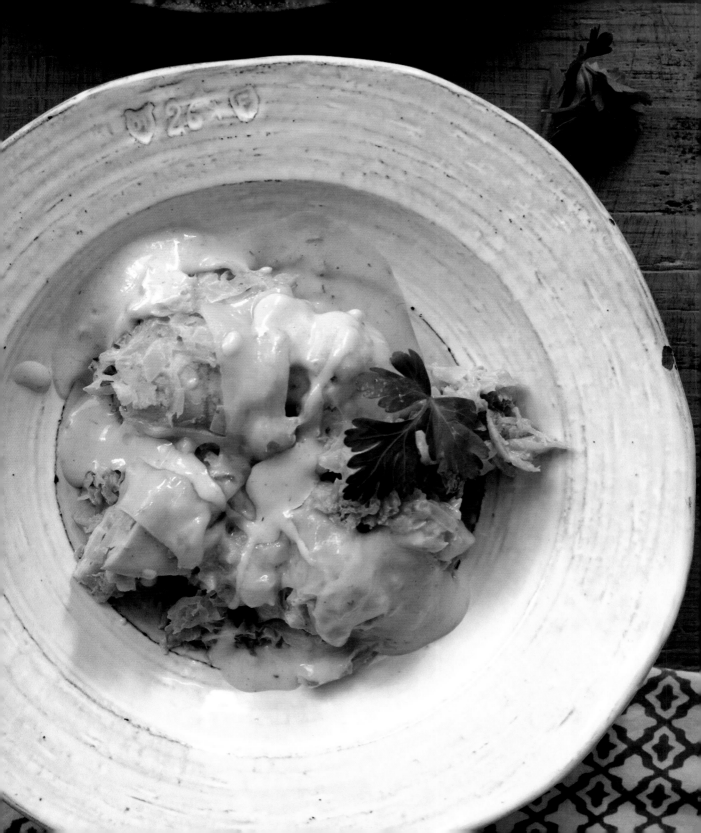

Chicken Reuben Bake

Gail Bush, Landenberg, PA

Makes 6 servings

Prep. Time: 10 minutes ⚜ Cooking Time: 6–8 hours ⚜ Setting: Slow Cook

4 boneless, skinless chicken-breast halves

¼ cup water

1-pound bag sauerkraut, drained and rinsed

4–5 (1 ounce each) slices Swiss cheese

¾ cup fat-free Thousand Island salad dressing

2 tablespoons chopped fresh parsley

1. Place chicken and water in inner pot of the Instant Pot along with ¼ cup water. Layer sauerkraut over chicken. Add cheese. Top with salad dressing. Sprinkle with parsley.

2. Secure the lid and cook on the Slow Cook setting on low 6–8 hours.

Exchange List Values

Carbohydrate 1.0
Meat—very lean 4.0

Basic Nutritional Values

Calories 217 (Calories from Fat 41)
Total Fat 5 gm (Saturated Fat 2.0 gm, Polyunsat Fat 0.6 gm, Monounsat Fat 1.4 gm)

Cholesterol 63 mg
Sodium 693 mg
Total Carb 13 gm
Dietary Fiber 2 gm
Sugars 6 gm
Protein 28 gm

Creamy Nutmeg Chicken

Amber Swarey, Donalds, SC

Makes 6 servings

Prep. Time: 20 minutes ♣ Cooking Time: 10 minutes ♣ Setting: Sauté and Manual
Pressure: High ♣ Release: Natural

1 tablespoon canola oil

6 boneless chicken breast halves, skin and visible fat removed

¼ cup chopped onion

¼ cup minced parsley

2 (10¾-ounce) cans 98% fat-free, reduced-sodium cream of mushroom soup

½ cup fat-free sour cream

½ cup fat-free milk

1 tablespoon ground nutmeg

¼ teaspoon sage

¼ teaspoon dried thyme

¼ teaspoon crushed rosemary

1. Press the Sauté button on the Instant Pot and then add the canola oil. Place the chicken in the oil and brown chicken on both sides. Remove the chicken to a plate.

2. Sauté the onion and parsley in the remaining oil in the Instant Pot until the onions are tender. Press Cancel on the Instant Pot, then place the chicken back inside.

3. Mix together the remaining ingredients in a bowl then pour over the chicken.

4. Secure the lid and set the vent to sealing. Set on Manual mode for 10 minutes.

5. When cooking time is up, let the pressure release naturally.

Exchange List Values

Carbohydrate 1.0
Meat—very lean 4.0
Fat 1.0

Basic Nutritional Values

Calories 264 (Calories from Fat 69)
Total Fat 8 gm (Saturated Fat 1.9 gm, Polyunsat Fat 2.1 gm, Monounsat Fat 2.8 gm)

Cholesterol 83 mg
Sodium 495 mg
Total Carb 15 gm
Dietary Fiber 1 gm
Sugars 5 gm
Protein 31 gm

Chicken in Mushroom Gravy

Rosemarie Fitzgerald, Gibsonia, PA
Audrey L. Kneer, WIlliamsfield, IL

Makes 6 servings
Prep. Time: 10 minutes & Cooking Time: 10 minutes & Setting: Manual
Pressure: High & Release: Natural

6 (5 ounces each) boneless, skinless chicken-breast halves

Salt and pepper to taste

¼ cup dry white wine or low-sodium chicken broth

10¾-ounce can 98% fat-free, reduced-sodium cream of mushroom soup

4 ounces sliced mushrooms

1. Place chicken in the inner pot of the Instant Pot. Season with salt and pepper.

2. Combine wine and soup in a bowl, then pour over the chicken. Top with the mushrooms.

3. Secure the lid and make sure the vent is set to sealing. Set on Manual mode for 10 minutes.

4. When cooking time is up, let the pressure release naturally.

Exchange List Values

Carbohydrate 0.5
Meat—very lean 4.0
Fat 0.5

Basic Nutritional Values

Calories 204 (Calories from Fat 40)
Total Fat 4 gm (Saturated Fat 1.4 gm, Polyunsat Fat 1.0 gm, Monounsat Fat 1.3 gm)

Cholesterol 85 mg
Sodium 320 mg
Total Carb 6 gm
Dietary Fiber 1 gm
Sugars 1 gm
Protein 34 gm

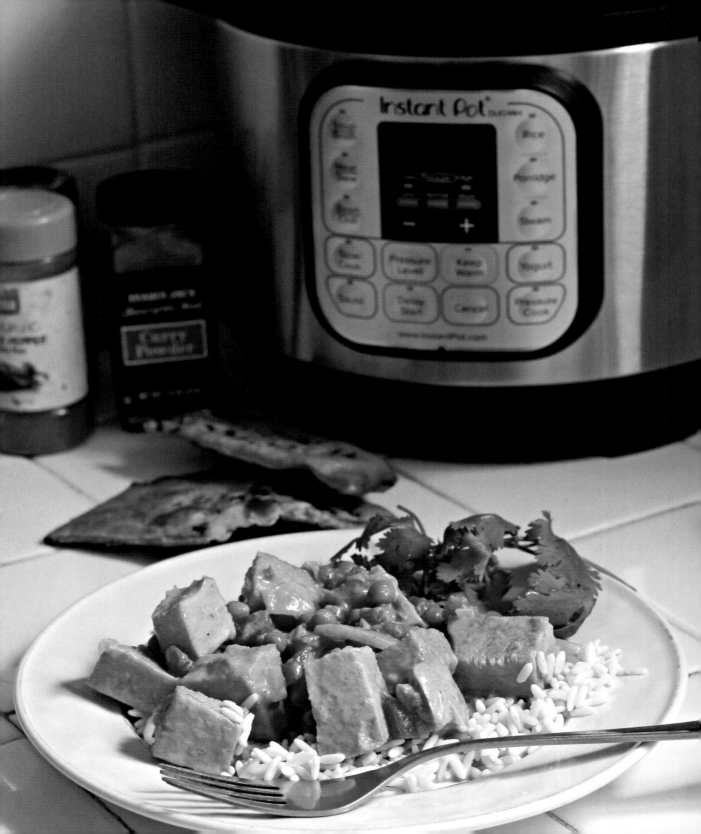

Mild Chicken Curry with Coconut Milk

Brittney Horst, Lititz, PA

Makes 4–6 servings
Prep. Time: 10 minutes ⚜ Cooking Time: 14 minutes ⚜ Setting: Sauté and Manual
Pressure: High ⚜ Release: Natural

1 large onion, diced

6 cloves garlic, crushed

¼ cup coconut oil

½ teaspoon black pepper

½ teaspoon turmeric

½ teaspoon paprika

¼ teaspoon cinnamon

¼ teaspoon cloves

¼ teaspoon cumin

¼ teaspoon ginger

½ teaspoon salt

1 tablespoon curry powder (more if you like more flavor)

½ teaspoon chili powder

24-ounce can of low-sodium diced or crushed tomatoes

13½-ounce can of light coconut milk (I prefer a brand that has no unwanted ingredients, like guar gum or sugar)

4 pounds boneless skinless chicken breasts, cut into chunks

Serving suggestion:
We like it on rice, with a couple of veggies on the side.

1. Sauté onion and garlic in the coconut oil, either with Sauté setting in the inner pot of the Instant Pot or on stove top, then add to pot.

2. Combine spices in a small bowl, then add to the inner pot.

3. Add tomatoes and coconut milk and stir.

4. Add chicken, and stir to coat the pieces with the sauce.

5. Secure the lid and make sure vent is at sealing. Set to Manual mode (or Pressure Cook on newer models) for 14 minutes.

6. Let pressure release naturally (if you're crunched for time, you can do a quick release).

7. Serve with your favorite sides, and enjoy!

Exchange List Values

Milk—skim 1.0
Fat 2.0
Meat—lean 1.0

Basic Nutritional Values

Calories 535 (Calories from Fat 189)
Total Fat 21 gm (Saturated Fat 12 gm, Polyunsat Fat 1.5 gm, Monounsat Fat 2.7 gm)

Cholesterol 221 mg
Sodium 315 mg
Total Carb 10 gm
Dietary Fiber 2.5 gm
Sugars 5 gm
Protein 71 gm

Turkey Meatballs and Gravy

Betty Sue Good, Broadway, VA

Makes 10 servings
Prep. Time: 35 minutes & Cooking Time: 10 minutes & Setting: Sauté and Manual
Pressure: High & Release: Natural

2 eggs, beaten

¾ cup bread crumbs

½ cup finely chopped onion

½ cup finely chopped celery

2 tablespoons chopped fresh parsley

¼ teaspoon pepper

⅛ teaspoon garlic powder

1½ pounds ground turkey

1½ tablespoons canola oil

10¾-ounce can 99% fat-free, reduced-sodium cream of mushroom soup

1 cup water

⅞-ounce package turkey gravy mix

½ teaspoon dried thyme

2 bay leaves

1. Combine eggs, bread crumbs, onion, celery, parsley, pepper, garlic powder, and meat. Shape into ¾" balls.

2. Set the Instant Pot to Sauté and add in the oil. Lightly brown meatballs in the oil in as many batches as needed. As the meatballs are browned, let them drain on a paper towel–lined plate or dish, then pat dry.

3. When all the meatballs are browned, press Cancel on the Instant Pot and then wipe out the inside of the inner pot. Place the meatballs back inside.

4. Combine soup, water, dry gravy mix, thyme, and bay leaves in a bowl, then pour over the meatballs.

5. Secure the lid and make sure the vent is set to sealing. Press the Manual button and set for 10 minutes.

6. When cook time is up, let the pressure release naturally. Discard bay leaves before serving.

Serving Suggestion:
Serve over mashed potatoes or buttered noodles.

Exchange List Values	Basic Nutritional Values	
Starch 0.5	Calories 212 (Calories from Fat 97)	Cholesterol 94 mg
Carbohydrate 0.5		Sodium 365 mg
Meat—lean 2.0	Total Fat 11 gm	Total Carb 11 gm
Fat 0.5	(Saturated Fat 2.5 gm, Polyunsat Fat 2.7 gm, Monounsat Fat 4.4 gm)	Dietary Fiber 1 gm
		Sugars 2 gm
		Protein 17 gm

Pizza in a Pot

Marianne J. Troyer, Millersburg, OH

Makes 8 servings

Prep. Time: 25 minutes ⚜ Cooking Time: 15 minutes ⚜ Setting: Sauté and Manual
Pressure: High ⚜ Release: Natural then Manual

1 pound bulk lean sweet Italian turkey sausage, browned and drained

28-ounce can crushed tomatoes

15½-ounce can chili beans

2¼-ounce can sliced black olives, drained

1 medium onion, chopped

1 small green bell pepper, chopped

2 garlic cloves, minced

¼ cup grated Parmesan cheese

1 tablespoon quick-cooking tapioca

1 tablespoon dried basil

1 bay leaf

1. Set the Instant Pot to Sauté, then add the turkey sausage. Sauté until browned.

2. Add the remaining ingredients into the Instant Pot and stir.

3. Secure the lid and make sure the vent is set to sealing. Cook on Manual for 15 minutes.

4. When cook time is up, let the pressure release naturally for 5 minutes then perform a quick release. Discard bay leaf.

Serving Suggestion:

Serve over pasta. Top with mozzarella cheese.

Exchange List Values

Starch 1.0
Vegetable 2.0
Meat—lean 2.0
Fat 0.5

Basic Nutritional Values

Calories 251 (Calories from Fat 87)
Total Fat 10 gm (Saturated Fat 2.8 gm, Polyunsat Fat 1.1 gm, Monounsat Fat 2.3 gm)

Cholesterol 49 mg
Sodium 937 mg
Total Carb 23 gm
Dietary Fiber 7 gm
Sugars 8 gm
Protein 18 gm

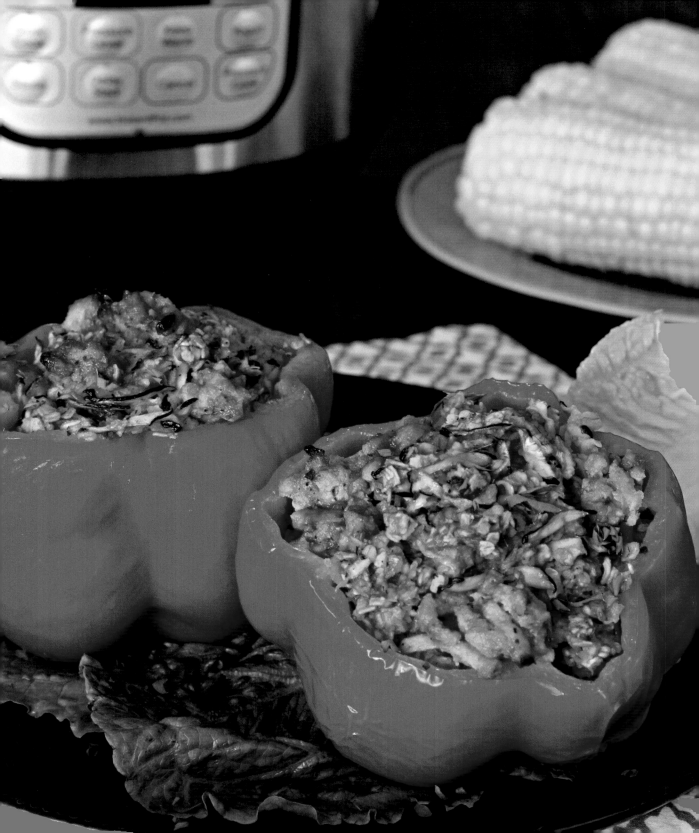

Taylor's Favorite Uniquely Stuffed Peppers

Maria Shevlin, Sicklerville, NJ

Makes 4 servings
Prep. Time: 20–30 minutes ⚜ Cooking Time: 15 minutes ⚜ Setting: Manual
Pressure: High ⚜ Release: Manual

4 red bell peppers
1 teaspoon olive oil
½ onion, chopped
3 cloves garlic, minced
½ pound ground turkey
½ pound spicy Italian sausage
1 teaspoon salt
½ teaspoons black pepper
1 teaspoon garlic powder
½ teaspoon dried oregano
½ teaspoon dried basil
1 medium zucchini, grated and water pressed out
½ cup of your favorite low-sugar barbecue sauce
¼ cup quick oats
1 cup water or low-sodium bone broth

1. Cut the stem part of the top off the bell peppers, remove seeds and membranes, and set aside.

2. Add olive oil, onion, and garlic to a pan. Cook till al dente.

3. Add ground turkey and sausage, and brown lightly.

4. Add seasonings, zucchini, and barbecue sauce.

5. Add oats.

6. Mix well to combine.

7. Stuff the filling inside each pepper—pack it in.

8. Add 1 cup of water or bone broth to the bottom of the inner pot of the Instant Pot.

9. Add the rack to the pot.

10. Arrange the stuffed peppers standing upright.

11. Lock lid, make sure vent is at sealing, and use the Manual setting to set for 15 minutes.

12. When cook time is up, release the pressure manually.

Exchange List Values

Vegetable 2.0
Fat 0.5
Meat—lean 1.0

Basic Nutritional Values

Calories 279 (Calories from Fat 63)
Total Fat 7 gm (Saturated Fat 1.8 gm, Polyunsat Fat 0.4 gm, Monounsat Fat 1.0 gm)
Cholesterol 72 mg
Sodium 1153 mg
Total Carb 28 gm
Dietary Fiber 4 gm
Sugars 17 gm
Protein 26 gm

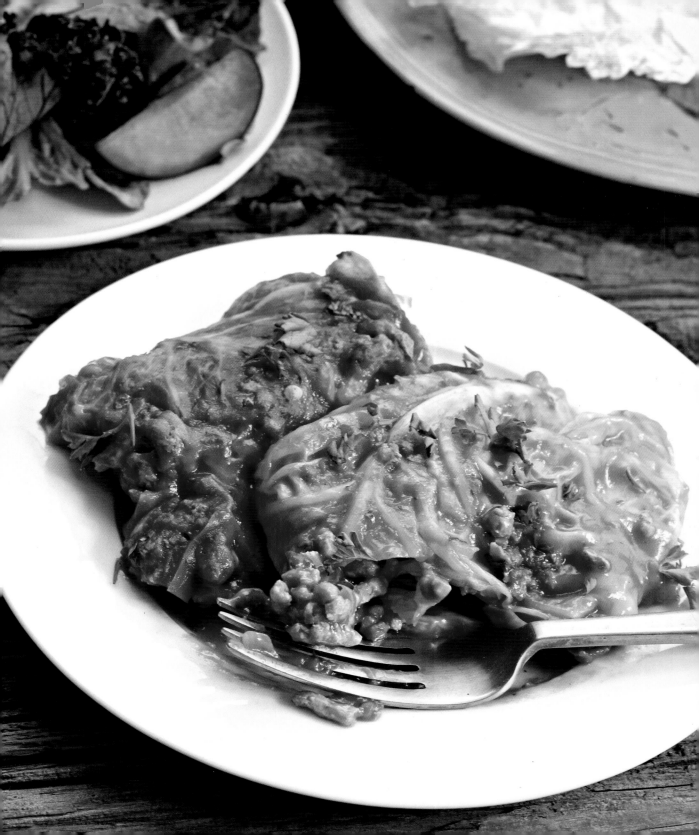

Cheesy Stuffed Cabbage

Maria Shevlin, Sicklerville, NJ

Makes 6–8 servings
Prep. Time: 30 minutes & Cooking Time: 18 minutes & Setting: Manual
Pressure: High & Release: Manual

1–2 heads savoy cabbage

1 pound ground turkey

1 egg

1 cup reduced-fat shredded cheddar cheese

2 tablespoons evaporated skim milk

¼ cup reduced-fat shredded Parmesan cheese

¼ cup reduced-fat shredded mozzarella cheese

¼ cup finely diced onion

¼ cup finely diced bell pepper

¼ cup finely diced mushrooms

1 teaspoon salt

½ teaspoon black pepper

1 teaspoon garlic powder

6 basil leaves, fresh and cut chiffonade

1 tablespoon fresh parsley, chopped

1 quart of your favorite pasta sauce

1. Remove the core from the cabbages.

2. Boil pot of water and place 1 head at a time into the water for approximately 10 minutes.

3. Allow cabbage to cool slightly. Once cooled, remove the leaves carefully and set aside. You'll need about 15 or 16.

4. Mix together the meat and all remaining ingredients except the pasta sauce.

5. One leaf at a time, put a heaping tablespoon of meat mixture in the center.

6. Tuck the sides in and then roll tightly.

7. Add ½ cup sauce to the bottom of the inner pot of the Instant Pot.

8. Place the rolls, fold-side down, into the pot and layer them, putting a touch of sauce between each layer and finally on top. (You may want to cook the rolls in two batches.)

9. Lock lid and make sure vent is at sealing. Set timer on 18 minutes on Manual at high pressure, then manually release the pressure when cook time is over.

Exchange List Values

Starch 1.5

Fat 0.5

Meat—lean 2.0

Vegetable 1.0

Basic Nutritional Values

Calories 199 (Calories from Fat 72)

Total Fat 8 gm (Saturated Fat 2.1 gm, Polyunsat Fat 0.2 gm, Monounsat Fat 0.4 gm)

Cholesterol 57 mg

Sodium 678 mg

Total Carb 14 gm

Dietary Fiber 3 gm

Sugars 7 gm

Protein 20 gm

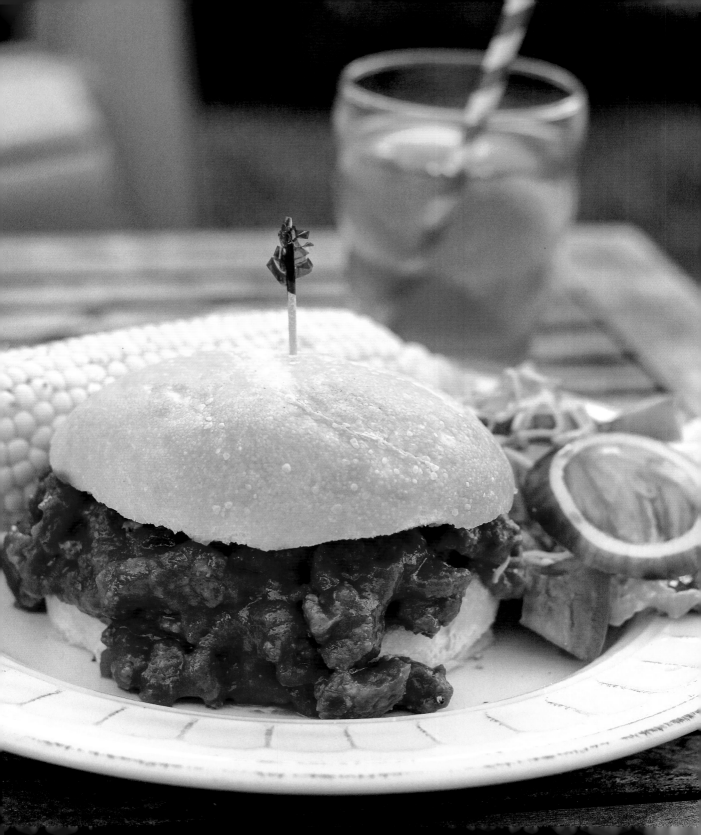

Turkey Sloppy Joes

Marla Folkerts, Holland, OH

Makes 6 servings
Prep. Time: 20 minutes ⚹ Cooking Time: 4 minutes ⚹ Setting: Sauté and Manual
Pressure: High ⚹ Release: Natural then Manual

I tablespoon olive oil

I red onion, chopped

I bell pepper, chopped

1½ pounds boneless turkey, finely chopped

I cup no-salt-added ketchup

½ teaspoons salt

I garlic clove, minced

I teaspoon Dijon-style mustard

⅛ teaspoon pepper

6 (1½ ounces each) multigrain sandwich rolls

1. Set the Instant Pot to Sauté and add the olive oil. Once the olive oil is hot, add in the onion, pepper and turkey. Sauté until the turkey is brown. Press Cancel.

2. Combine ketchup, salt, garlic, mustard, and pepper, then pour over the turkey mixture. Mix well.

3. Secure the lid and make sure the vent is set to sealing. Put the Instant Pot on Manual mode for 15 minutes.

4. When cook time is up, let the pressure release naturally for 5 minutes, then perform a quick release. Serve on homemade bread or sandwich rolls.

Exchange List Values

Starch 2.0

Fat 0.5

Meat—lean 1

Basic Nutritional Values

Calories 296 (Calories from Fat 63)

Total Fat 7 gm (Saturated Fat 0.7 gm, Polyunsat Fat 1.0 gm, Monounsat Fat 2.3 gm)

Cholesterol 60 mg

Sodium 432 mg

Total Carb 27 gm

Dietary Fiber 3 gm

Sugars 13 gm

Protein 33 gm

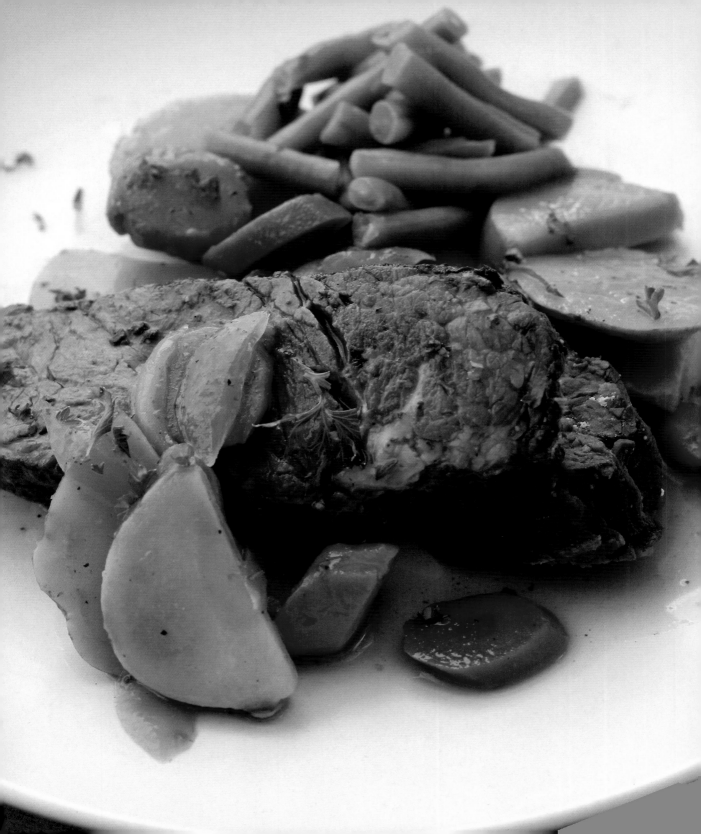

Pot Roast

Carole Whaling, New Tripoli, PA

Makes 8 servings
Prep. Time: 20 minutes ⚜ Cooking Time: 35 minutes ⚜ Setting: Sauté and Manual
Pressure: High ⚜ Release: Natural

2 tablespoons olive oil

3–4 pound rump roast, or pot roast, bone removed, and cut into serving-sized pieces, trimmed of fat

4 medium potatoes, cubed or sliced

4 medium carrots, sliced

I medium onion, sliced

I teaspoon salt

½ teaspoon pepper

I cup low-sodium beef broth

1. Press the Sauté button on the Instant Pot and add the olive oil. Once the oil is heated, lightly brown the pieces of roast, about 2 minutes on each side. Press Cancel.

2. Leave roast in Instant Pot and add the veggies around it around the roast, along with the salt, pepper and beef broth.

3. Secure the lid and make sure the vent is set to sealing. Set the Instant Pot to Manual mode for 35 minutes. Let pressure release naturally when cook time is up.

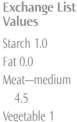

Exchange List Values

Starch 1.0

Fat 0.0

Meat—medium
    4.5

Vegetable 1

Basic Nutritional Values

Calories 394 (Calories from Fat 189)

Total Fat 21 gm
    (Saturated Fat 7.6 gm, Polyunsat Fat 1.1 gm, Monounsat Fat 10.3 gm)

Cholesterol 105 mg

Sodium 368 mg

Total Carb 12 gm

Dietary Fiber 2 gm

Sugars 2 gm

Protein 36 gm

Pot Roast with Tomato Sauce

Carol Eveleth, Cheyenne, WY

Makes 4–6 servings
Prep. Time: 20 minutes ⚭ Cooking Time: 2 hours ⚭ Setting: Manual
Pressure: High ⚭ Release: Manual

2 pounds beef roast, boneless

¼ teaspoon salt

¼ teaspoon pepper

1 tablespoon olive oil

2 stalks celery, chopped

4 tablespoons margarine

2 cups low-sodium tomato juice

2 cloves garlic, finely chopped, or 1 teaspoon garlic powder

1 teaspoon thyme

1 bay leaf

4 carrots, chopped

1 medium onion, chopped

4 medium potatoes, chopped

1. Pat beef dry with paper towels; season on all sides with salt and pepper.

2. Select Sauté function on the Instant Pot and adjust heat to more. Put the oil in the inner pot, then cook the beef in oil for 6 minutes, until browned, turning once. Set on plate.

3. Add celery and margarine to the inner pot; cook 2 minutes. Stir in tomato juice, garlic, thyme, and bay leaf. Hit Cancel to turn off Sauté function.

4. Place beef on top of the contents of the inner pot and press into sauce. Cover and lock lid and make sure vent is at sealing. Select Manual and cook at high pressure for 1 hour 15 minutes.

5. Once cooking is complete, release pressure by using natural release function. Transfer beef to cutting board. Discard bay leaf.

6. Skim off any excess fat from surface. Choose Sauté function and adjust heat to more. Cook 18 minutes, or until reduced by about half (2½ cups). Hit Cancel to turn off Sauté function.

7. Add carrots, onion, and potatoes. Cover and lock lid and make sure vent is at sealing. Select Manual and cook at high pressure for 10 minutes.

8. Once cooking is complete, release pressure by using a quick release. Using Sauté function, keep at a simmer.

9. Season with more salt and pepper to taste.

Serving suggestion:

Brighten this dish up with some colorful, freshly steamed broccoli when serving.

Exchange List Values	Basic Nutritional Values	
Starch 2.5	Calories 391 (Calories from Fat 171)	Cholesterol 104 mg
Fat 0.5		Sodium 395 mg
Meat—medium 3.5	Total Fat 19 gm (Saturated Fat 5.7 gm, Polyunsat Fat 3.1 gm, Monounsat Fat 10 gm)	Total Carb 22 gm
Vegetable 1.5		Dietary Fiber 4 gm
		Sugars 6 gm
		Protein 34 gm

Pot Roast with Gravy and Vegetables

Irene Klaeger, Inverness, FL
Jan Pembleton, Arlington, TX

Makes 6 servings
Prep. Time: 30 minutes ⚘ *Cooking Time: 1 hour 15 minutes* ⚘ *Setting: Sauté and Manual*
Pressure: High ⚘ *Release: Natural*

1 tablespoon olive oil

3–4 pound bottom round, rump, or arm roast, trimmed of fat

¼ teaspoon salt

2–3 teaspoons pepper

2 tablespoons flour

1 cup cold water

1 teaspoon Kitchen Bouquet, or gravy browning seasoning sauce

1 garlic clove, minced

2 medium onions, cut in wedges

4 medium potatoes, cubed, unpeeled

2 carrots, quartered

1 green bell pepper, sliced

1. Press the Sauté button on the Instant Pot and pour the oil inside, letting it heat up. Sprinkle each side of the roast with salt and pepper, then brown it for 5 minutes on each side inside the pot.

2. Mix together the flour, water and Kitchen Bouquet and spread over roast.

3. Add garlic, onions, potatoes, carrots, and green pepper.

4. Secure the lid and make sure the vent is set to sealing. Press Manual and set the Instant Pot for 1 hour and 15 minutes.

5. When cook time is up, let the pressure release naturally.

Exchange List Values

Starch 2.0
Fat 0.0
Meat—medium fat 6
Vegetable 1

Basic Nutritional Values

Calories 551 (Calories from Fat 270)
Total Fat 30 gm (Saturated Fat 11 gm, Polyunsat Fat 1.4 gm, Monounsat Fat 13.5 gm)

Cholesterol 170 mg
Sodium 256 mg
Total Carb 19 gm
Dietary Fiber 3.2 gm
Sugars 2.7 gm
Protein 49 gm

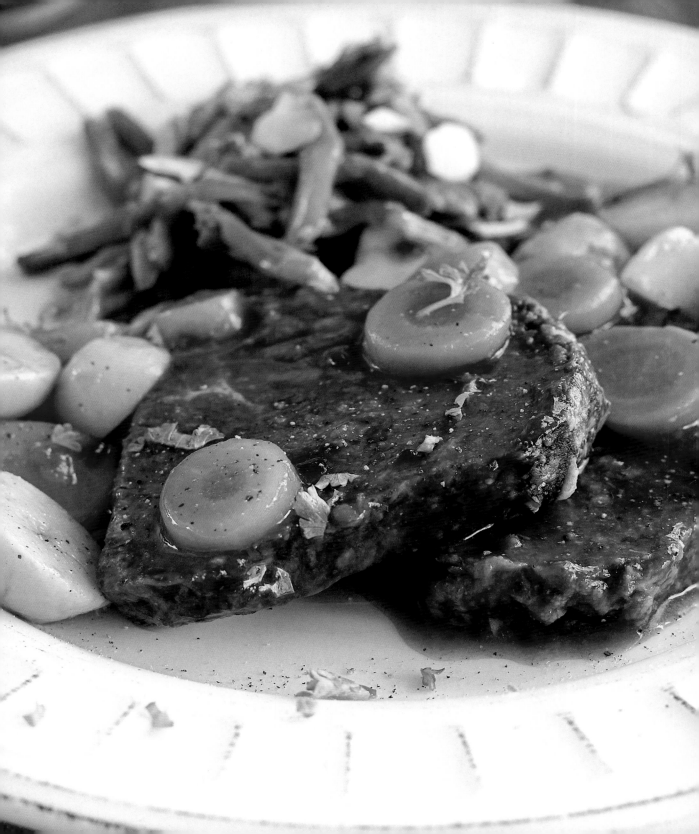

Easy Pot Roast and Vegetables

Tina Houk, Clinton, MO
Arlene Wines, Newton, KS

Makes 6 servings
Prep. Time: 20 minutes ☙ Cooking Time: 35 minutes ☙ Setting: Manual
Pressure: High ☙ Release: Natural

3–4 pound chuck roast, trimmed of fat and cut into serving-sized chunks

4 medium potatoes, cubed, unpeeled

4 medium carrots, sliced, or 1 pound baby carrots

2 celery ribs, sliced thin

1 envelope dry onion soup mix

3 cups water

1. Place the pot roast chunks and vegetables into the Instant Pot along with the potatoes, carrots and celery.

2. Mix together the onion soup mix and water and pour over the contents of the Instant Pot.

3. Secure the lid and make sure the vent is set to sealing. Set the Instant Pot to Manual mode for 35 minutes. Let pressure release naturally when cook time is up.

Variation:

Before putting roast in cooker, sprinkle it with the dry soup mix, patting it on so it adheres.

—Betty Lahman, Elkton, VA

Exchange List Values

Starch 1.5
Vegetable 1.0
Meat—lean 3.0

Basic Nutritional Values

Calories 325 (Calories from Fat 76)
Total Fat 8 gm (Saturated Fat 2.9 gm, Polyunsat Fat 0.5 gm, Monounsat Fat 3.6 gm)

Cholesterol 98 mg
Sodium 560 mg
Total Carb 26 gm
Dietary Fiber 4 gm
Sugars 6 gm
Protein 35 gm

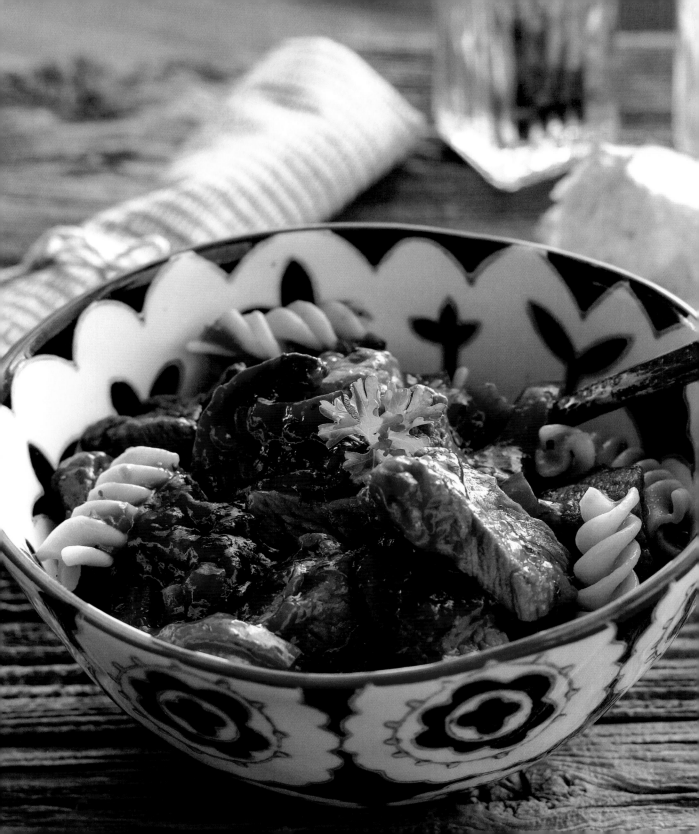

Beef Burgundy

Jacqueline Stefl, East Bethany, NY

Makes 6 servings
Prep. Time: 30 minutes ⚹ Cooking Time: 30 minutes ⚹ Setting: Sauté and Manual
Pressure: High ⚹ Release: Natural then Manual

2 tablespoons olive oil

2 pounds stewing meat, cubed, trimmed of fat

2½ tablespoons flour

5 medium onions, thinly sliced

½ pound fresh mushrooms, sliced

1 teaspoon salt

¼ teaspoon dried marjoram

¼ teaspoon dried thyme

⅛ teaspoon pepper

¾ cup beef broth

1½ cups burgundy

1. Press Sauté on the Instant pot and add in the olive oil.

2. Dredge meat in flour, then brown in batches in the Instant Pot. Set aside the meat. Sauté the onions and mushrooms in the remaining oil and drippings for about 3–4 minutes, then add the meat back in. Press Cancel.

3. Add the salt, marjoram, thyme, pepper, broth, and wine to the Instant Pot.

4. Secure the lid and make sure the vent is set to sealing. Press the Manual button and set to 30 minutes.

5. When cook time is up, let the pressure release naturally for 15 minutes, then perform a quick release.

6. Serve over cooked noodles.

Exchange List Values

Meat—lean 5.5
Fat 0.0

Basic Nutritional Values

Calories 358 (Calories from Fat 1)
Total Fat 11 gm
(Saturated Fat 3 gm, Polyunsat Fat 0.9 gm, Monounsat Fat 6.5 gm)

Cholesterol 80 mg
Sodium 472 mg
Total Carb 15 gm
Dietary Fiber 2 gm
Sugars 5 gm
Protein 37 gm

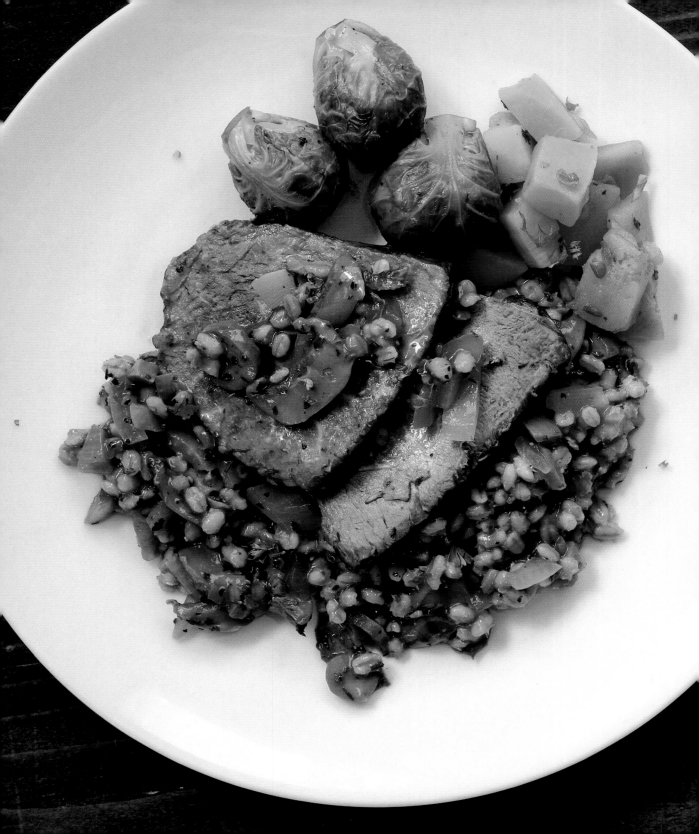

Beef Roast with Mushroom Barley

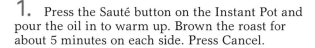

Sue Hamilton, Minooka, IL

Makes 6 servings

Prep. Time: 20 minutes ⚜ Cooking Time: 1 hour 15 minutes ⚜ Setting: Sauté and Manual
Pressure: High ⚜ Release: Natural and Manual

1 tablespoon olive oil

2-pound beef chuck roast, visible fat removed

1 cup pearl barley (not quick-cook)

½ cup onion, diced

6½-ounce can mushrooms, undrained

1 teaspoon minced garlic

1 teaspoon Italian seasoning

¼ teaspoon black pepper

1¾ cups beef broth

1. Press the Sauté button on the Instant Pot and pour the oil in to warm up. Brown the roast for about 5 minutes on each side. Press Cancel.

2. Add the rest of the ingredients to the Instant Pot, then secure the lid, making sure the vent is set to sealing.

3. Press the Manual button and set the time for 1 hour and 15 minutes.

4. When cook time is up, let the pressure release naturally for 15 minutes, then perform a quick release.

Serving Suggestion:

Serve this with mashed potatoes. They'll benefit from the delicious broth in this dish.

Exchange List Values

Starch 3.0
Fat 0.5
Meat—lean 3.5
Vegetable 15

Basic Nutritional Values

Calories 353 (Calories from Fat 108)
Total Fat 12 gm
(Saturated Fat 4 gm, Polyunsat Fat 1.0 gm, Monounsat Fat 6.2 gm)

Cholesterol 101 mg
Sodium 354 mg
Total Carb 25 gm
Dietary Fiber 6 gm
Sugars 1 gm
Protein 37 gm

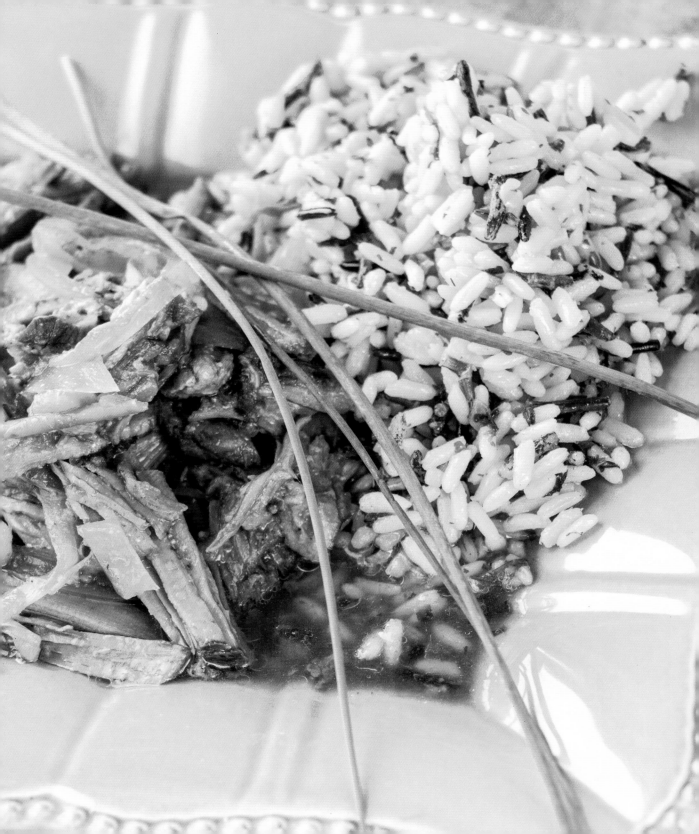

Machaca Beef

Jeanne Allen, Rye, CO

Makes 12 servings
Prep. Time: 15 minutes ☙ Cooking Time: 10–12 hours ☙ Setting: Slow Cook

1½-pound beef roast
1 large onion, sliced
4-ounce can chopped green chilies
2 beef bouillon cubes
1½ teaspoons dry mustard
½ teaspoon garlic powder
1 teaspoon seasoning salt
½ teaspoon pepper
1 cup water
1 cup salsa

1. Combine all ingredients except salsa in the Instant Pot inner pot.

2. Secure the lid and make sure the vent is set to sealing. Press the Slow Cook button and set on low for 12 hours, or until beef is tender. Drain and reserve liquid.

3. Shred beef using two forks to pull it apart.

4. Combine beef, salsa, and enough of the reserved liquid to make desired consistency.

5. Use this filling for burritos, chalupas, quesadillas, or tacos.

Exchange List Values

Meat—lean 1.0

Basic Nutritional Values

Calories 69 (Calories from Fat 20)
Total Fat 2 gm (Saturated Fat 0.7 gm, Polyunsat Fat 0.1 gm, Monounsat Fat 0.9 gm)

Cholesterol 24 mg
Sodium 392 mg
Total Carb 3 gm
Dietary Fiber 1 gm
Sugars 2 gm
Protein 9 gm

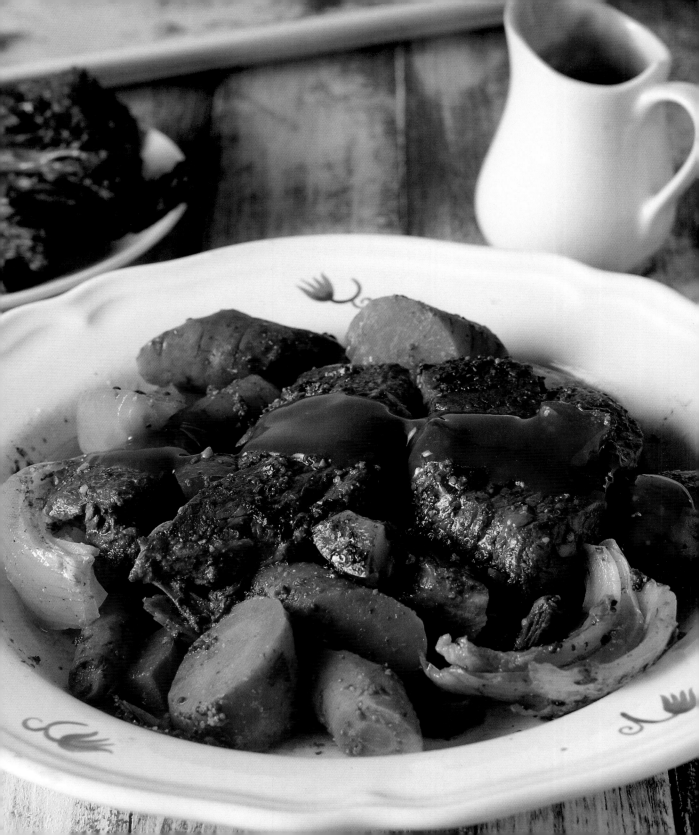

Bavarian Beef

Naomi E. Fast, Hesston, KS

Makes 8 servings
Prep. Time: 35 minutes & Cooking Time: 1 hour 15 minutes & Setting: Sauté and Manual
Pressure: High & Release: Natural

1 tablespoon canola oil

3-pound boneless beef chuck roast, trimmed of fat

3 cups sliced carrots

3 cups sliced onions

2 large kosher dill pickles, chopped

1 cup sliced celery

½ cup dry red wine or beef broth

⅓ cup German-style mustard

2 teaspoons coarsely ground black pepper

2 bay leaves

¼ teaspoon ground cloves

1 cup water

⅓ cup flour

1. Press Sauté on the Instant Pot and add in the oil. Brown roast on both sides for about 5 minutes. Press Cancel.

2. Add all of the remaining ingredients, except for the flour, to the Instant Pot.

3. Secure the lid and make sure the vent is set to sealing. Press Manual and set the time to 1 hour and 15 minutes. Let the pressure release naturally.

4. Remove meat and vegetables to large platter. Cover to keep warm.

5. Remove 1 cup of the liquid from the Instant Pot and mix with the flour. Press Sauté on the Instant Pot and add the flour/broth mixture back in, whisking. Cook until the broth is smooth and thickened.

6. Serve over noodles or spaetzle.

Exchange List Values

Starch 0.5
Vegetable 2.0
Meat—lean 3.0

Basic Nutritional Values

Calories 251 (Calories from Fat 76)
Total Fat 8 gm
(Saturated Fat 2.4 gm, Polyunsat Fat 0.9 gm, Monounsat Fat 3.8 gm)

Cholesterol 73 mg
Sodium 525 mg
Total Carb 17 gm
Dietary Fiber 4 gm
Sugars 7 gm
Protein 26 gm

Zesty Swiss Steak

Marilyn Mowry, Irving, TX

Makes 6 servings
Prep. Time: 35 minutes & Cooking Time: 35 minutes & Setting: Sauté and Manual
Pressure: High & Release: Natural then Manual

3–4 tablespoons flour

½ teaspoon salt

¼ teaspoon pepper

1½ teaspoons dry mustard

1½–2 pounds round steak, trimmed of fat

1 tablespoon canola oil

1 cup sliced onions

1 pound carrots, sliced

14½-ounce can whole tomatoes

⅓ cup water

1 tablespoon brown sugar

1½ tablespoons Worcestershire sauce

1. Combine flour, salt, pepper, and dry mustard.

2. Cut steak in serving pieces. Dredge in flour mixture.

3. Set the Instant Pot to Sauté and add in the oil. Brown the steak pieces on both sides in the oil. Press Cancel.

4. Add onions and carrots into the Instant Pot.

5. Combine the tomatoes, water, brown sugar, and Worcestershire sauce. Pour into the Instant Pot.

6. Secure the lid and make sure the vent is set to sealing. Press Manual and set the time for 35 minutes.

7. When cook time is up, let the pressure release naturally for 15 minutes, then perform a quick release.

Exchange List Values

Vegetable 3.0
Meat—lean 3.0

Basic Nutritional Values

Calories 236 (Calories from Fat 71)
Total Fat 8 gm
    (Saturated Fat 1.9 gm, Polyunsat Fat 1.0 gm, Monounsat Fat 3.6 gm)

Cholesterol 64 mg
Sodium 426 mg
Total Carb 18 gm
Dietary Fiber 3 gm
Sugars 9 gm
Protein 23 gm

Asian Pepper Steak

Donna Lantgen, Rapid City, SD

Makes 6 servings
Prep. Time: 20 minutes ⚘ Cooking Time: 6–8 hours ⚘ Setting: Slow Cook

I pound round steak, sliced thin, trimmed of fat

3 tablespoons light soy sauce

½ teaspoon ground ginger

I garlic clove, minced

I medium green pepper, thinly sliced

4-ounce can mushrooms, drained, or I cup sliced fresh mushrooms

I medium onion, thinly sliced

½ teaspoons crushed red pepper

1. Combine all ingredients in the inner pot of the Instant Pot.

2. Secure the lid and press Slow Cook on low 6–8 hours.

3. Serve as steak sandwiches topped with provolone cheese, or over rice.

Exchange List Values

Vegetable 1.0
Meat—lean 2.0

Basic Nutritional Values

Calories 122 (Calories from Fat 32)
Total Fat 4 gm
(Saturated Fat 1.2 gm, Polyunsat Fat 0.2 gm, Monounsat Fat 1.5 gm)
Cholesterol 43 mg
Sodium 368 mg
Total Carb 6 gm
Dietary Fiber 2 gm
Sugars 3 gm
Protein 16 gm

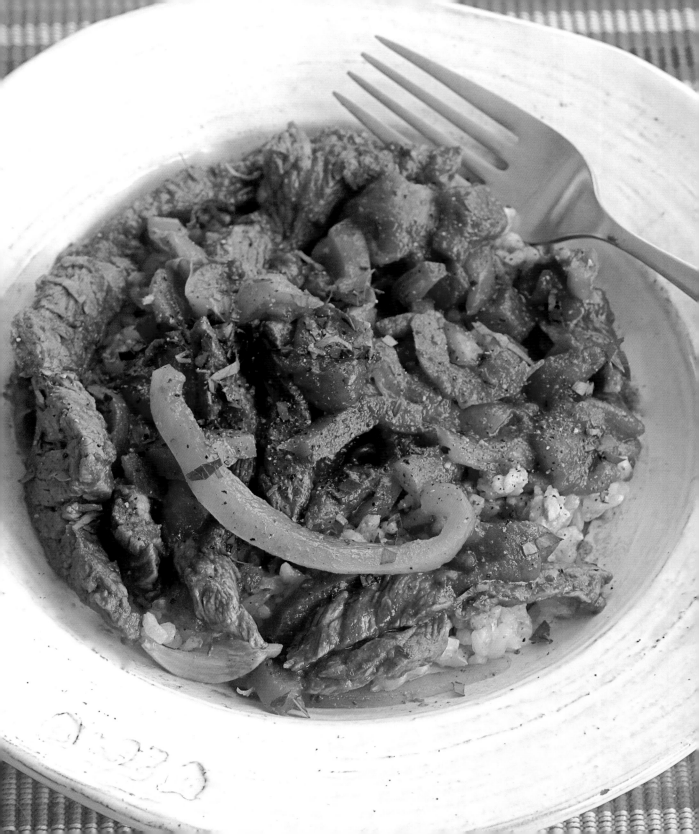

Three-Pepper Steak

Renee Hankins, Narvon, PA

Makes 10 servings
Prep. Time: 15 minutes ⚜ Cooking Time: 15 minutes ⚜ Setting: Manual
Pressure: High ⚜ Release: Natural then Manual

3-pound beef flank steak, cut in
¼-½"-thick slices across the grain

3 bell peppers—one red, one orange,
and one yellow pepper (or any
combination of colors), cut into
¼"-thick slices

2 garlic cloves, sliced

I large onion, sliced

I teaspoon ground cumin

½ teaspoon dried oregano

I bay leaf

¼ cup water

Salt to taste

14½-ounce can diced tomatoes in juice

Jalapeño chilies, sliced, *optional*

1. Place all ingredients into the Instant Pot and stir.

2. Sprinkle with jalapeño pepper slices if you wish.

3. Secure the lid and make sure vent is set to sealing. Press Manual and set the time for 15 minutes.

4. When cook time is up, let the pressure release naturally for 15 minutes, then perform a quick release of the remaining pressure.

Serving Suggestion:

We love this served over
noodles, rice, or torn tortillas.

Exchange List Values

Vegetable 1.0
Meat—lean 4.0

Basic Nutritional Values

Calories 220 (Calories
from Fat 70)
Total Fat 8 gm
(Saturated Fat 3.0
gm, Polyunsat Fat
0 gm Monounsat
Fat 2.5 gm)

Cholesterol 85 mg
Sodium 135 mg
Total Carb 7 gm
Dietary Fiber 1 gm
Sugars 3 gm
Protein 30 gm

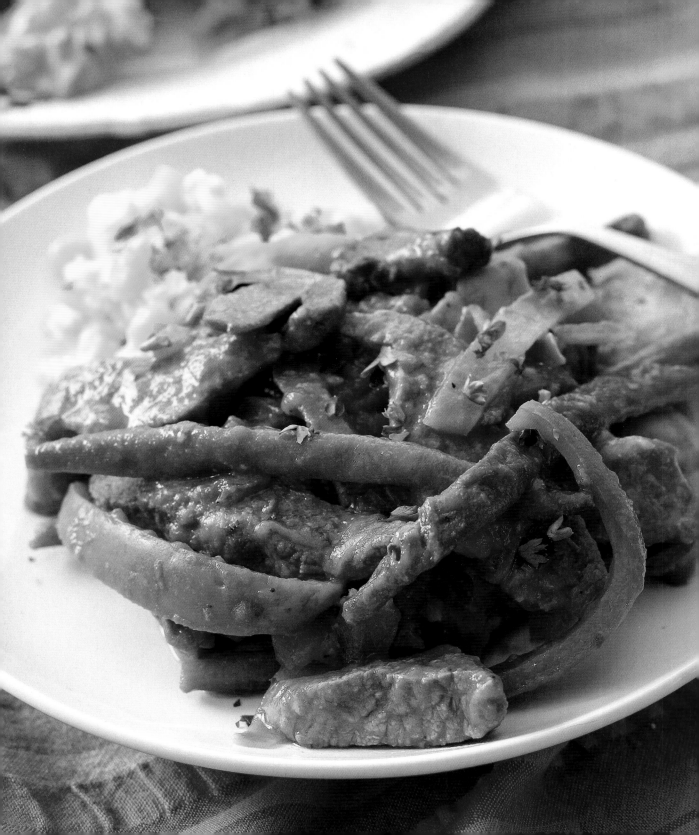

"Smothered" Steak

Susan Yoder Graber, Eureka, IL

Makes 6 servings
Prep. Time: 20 minutes ⚜ Cooking Time: 15 minutes ⚜ Setting: Sauté and Manual
Pressure: High ⚜ Release: Natural then Manual

1 tablespoon olive oil

¼ teaspoon pepper

⅓ cup flour

1½-pound chuck, or round, steak, cut into strips, trimmed of fat

1 large onion, sliced

1 green pepper, sliced

14½-ounce can stewed tomatoes

4-ounce can mushrooms, drained

2 tablespoons soy sauce

10-ounce package frozen French-style green beans

1. Press Sauté and add the oil to the Instant Pot.

2. Mix together the flour and pepper in a small bowl. Place the steak pieces into the mixture in the bowl and coat each of them well.

3. Lightly brown each of the steak pieces in the Instant Pot, about 2 minutes on each side. Press Cancel when done.

4. Add the remaining ingredients to the Instant Pot and mix together gently.

5. Secure the lid and make sure vent is set to sealing. Press Manual and set for 15 minutes.

6. When cook time is up, let the pressure release naturally for 15 minutes, then perform a quick release.

Serving suggestion:

Serve over rice.

Variations:

1. Use 8-ounce can tomato sauce instead of stewed tomatoes.

2. Substitute 1 tablespoon Worcestershire sauce in place of soy sauce.

—Mary E. Martin, Goshen, IN

Exchange List Values

Starch 2.0
Fat 2.5
Meat—medium 2.0
Vegetable 1.5

Basic Nutritional Values

Calories 386 (Calories from Fat 216)
Total Fat 24 gm (Saturated Fat 8.9 gm, Polyunsat Fat 1.7 gm, Monounsat Fat 11.5 gm)
Cholesterol 77 mg
Sodium 746 mg
Total Carb 20 gm
Dietary Fiber 4 gm
Sugars 4 gm
Protein 25 gm

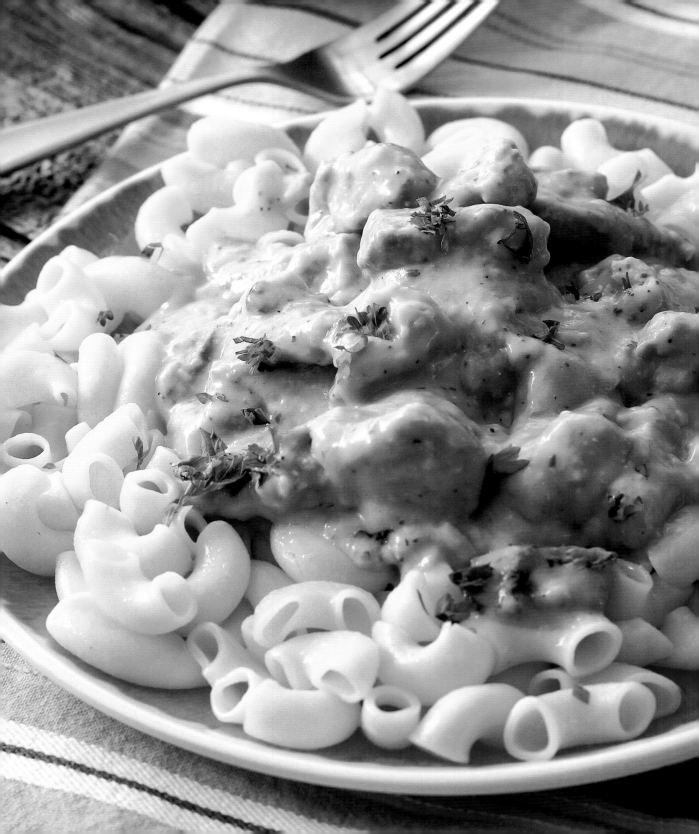

Steak Stroganoff

Marie Morucci, Glen Lyon, PA

Makes 6 servings
Prep. Time: 15 minutes ⚜ Cooking Time: 30 minutes ⚜ Setting: Sauté and Manual
Pressure: High ⚜ Release: Natural then Manual

1 tablespoon olive oil

2 tablespoons flour

½ teaspoon garlic powder

½ teaspoon pepper

¼ teaspoon paprika

1¾-pound boneless beef round steak, trimmed of fat, cut into 1½ × ½-inch strips.

10¾-ounce can reduced-sodium, 98% fat-free cream of mushroom soup

½ cup water

1 envelope sodium-free dried onion soup mix

9-ounces jar sliced mushrooms, drained

½ cup fat-free sour cream

1 tablespoon minced fresh parsley

1. Place the oil in the Instant Pot and press Sauté.

2. Combine flour, garlic powder, pepper, and paprika in a small bowl. Stir the steak pieces through the flour mixture until they are evenly coated.

3. Lightly brown the steak pieces in the oil in the Instant Pot, about 2 minutes each side. Press Cancel when done.

4. Stir the mushroom soup, water, and onion soup mix then pour over the steak.

5. Secure the lid and set the vent to sealing. Press the Manual button and set for 15 minutes.

6. When cook time is up, let the pressure release naturally for 15 minutes, then release the rest manually.

7. Remove the lid and press Cancel then Sauté. Stir in mushrooms, sour cream, and parsley. Let the sauce come to a boil and cook for about 10–15 minutes.

Exchange List Values

Meat—lean 5

Basic Nutritional Values

Calories 248 (Calories from Fat 54)
Total Fat 6 gm (Saturated Fat 1.7 gm, Polyunsat Fat 1.2 gm, Monounsat Fat 3.2 gm)
Cholesterol 68 mg
Sodium 563 mg
Total Carb 12 gm
Dietary Fiber 2 gm
Sugars 2 gm
Protein 33 gm

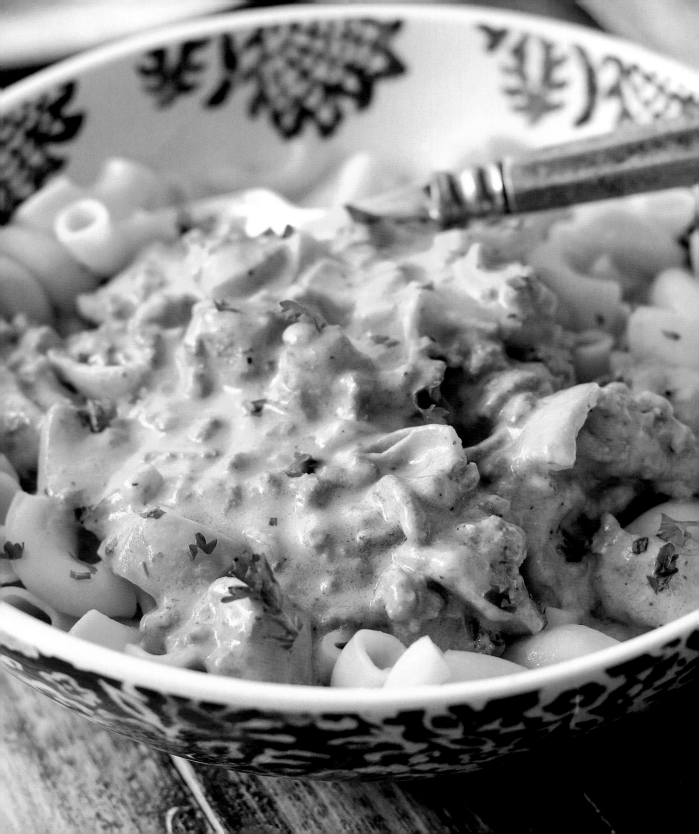

Garlic Beef Stroganoff

Sharon Miller, Holmesville, OH

Makes 6 servings
Prep. Time: 20 minutes ⚜ *Cooking Time: 25 minutes* ⚜ *Setting: Saute and Manual*
Pressure: High ⚜ *Release: Natural and Manual*

2 tablespoons canola oil

1½ pounds boneless round steak, cut into thin strips, trimmed of fat

2 teaspoons sodium-free beef bouillon powder

1 cup mushroom juice, with water added to make a full cup

2 (4½-ounce) jars sliced mushrooms, drained with juice reserved

10¾-ounce can 98% fat-free, lower-sodium cream of mushroom soup

1 large onion, chopped

3 garlic cloves, minced

1 tablespoon Worcestershire sauce

6-ounces fat-free cream cheese, cubed and softened

1. Press the Sauté button and put the oil into the Instant Pot inner pot.

2. Once the oil is heated, sauté the beef until it is lightly browned, about 2 minutes on each side. Set the beef aside for a moment. Press Cancel and wipe out the Instant Pot with some paper towel.

3. Press Sauté again and dissolve the bouillon in the mushroom juice and water in inner pot of the Instant Pot. Once dissolved, press Cancel.

4. Add the mushrooms, soup, onion, garlic, and Worcestershire sauce and stir. Add the beef back to the pot.

5. Secure the lid and make sure the vent is set to sealing. Press Manual and set for 15 minutes.

6. When cook time is up, let the pressure release naturally for 15 minutes, then perform a quick release.

7. Press Cancel and remove the lid. Press Sauté. Stir in cream cheese until smooth.

8. Serve over noodles.

Exchange List Values

Carbohydrate 0.5
Vegetable 1.0
Meat—lean 2.0
Fat 0.5

Basic Nutritional Values

Calories 202 (Calories from Fat 73)
Total Fat 8 gm
(Saturated Fat 1.8 gm, Polyunsat Fat 1.4 gm, Monounsat Fat 3.9 gm)

Cholesterol 51 mg
Sodium 474 mg
Total Carb 10 gm
Dietary Fiber 2 gm
Sugars 4 gm
Protein 21 gm

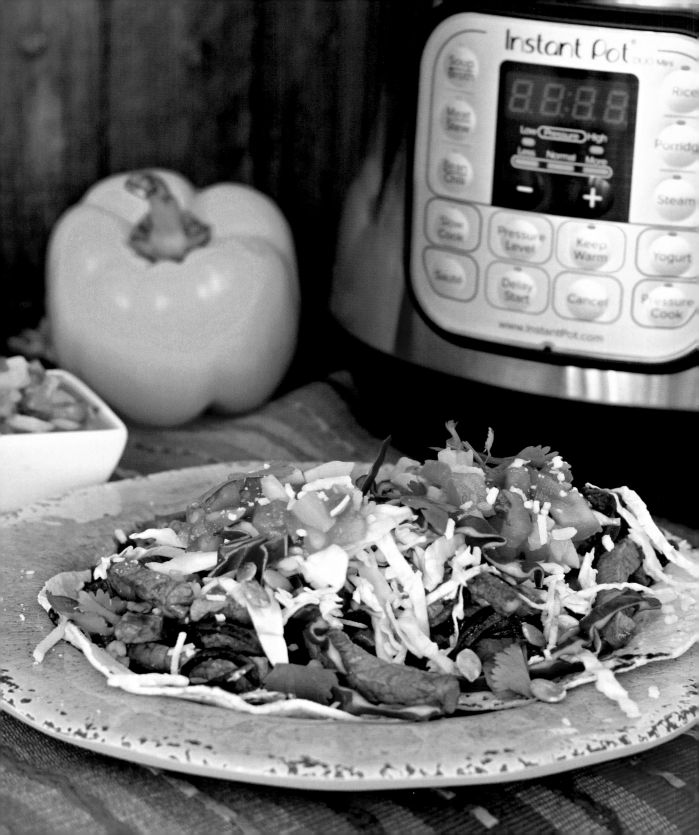

Quick Steak Tacos

Hope Comerford, Clinton Township, MI

Makes 6 servings
Prep. Time: 5 minutes ⚜ Cooking Time: 10 minutes ⚜ Setting: Sauté

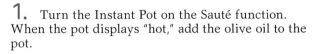

1 tablespoon olive oil
8 ounces sirloin steak
2 tablespoons steak seasoning
1 teaspoon Worcestershire sauce
½ red onion, halved and sliced
6 corn tortillas
¼ cup tomatoes
¾ cup reduced-fat Mexican cheese
2 tablespoons low-fat sour cream
6 tablespoons garden fresh salsa
¼ cup chopped fresh cilantro

1. Turn the Instant Pot on the Sauté function. When the pot displays "hot," add the olive oil to the pot.

2. Season the steak with the steak seasoning.

3. Add the steak to the pot along with the Worcestershire sauce.

4. Cook each side of the steak for 2–3 minutes until the steak turns brown.

5. Remove the steak from the pot and slice thinly.

6. Add the onion to the pot with the remaining olive oil and steak juices and cook them until translucent.

7. Remove the onion from the pot.

8. Warm your corn tortillas, then assemble your steak, onion, tomatoes, cheese, sour cream, salsa, and cilantro on top of each.

Exchange List Values

Starch 1.5
Fat 1.0
Meat—medium 1.0
Vegetable 1.0

Basic Nutritional Values

Calories 187 (Calories from Fat 81)
Total Fat 9 gm (Saturated Fat 3.8 gm, Polyunsat Fat 0.8 gm, Monounsat Fat 3.7 gm)
Cholesterol 40 mg
Sodium 254 mg
Total Carb 14 gm
Dietary Fiber 2 gm
Sugars 2 gm
Protein 14 gm

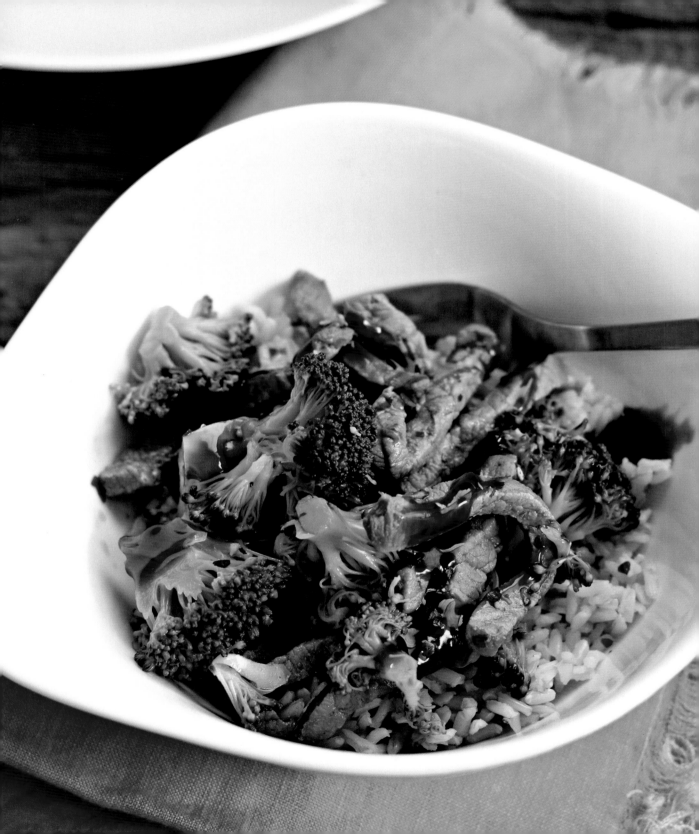

Beef Broccoli

Anita Troyer, Fairview, MI

Makes 6 servings
Prep. Time: 15 minutes   ♣   Cooking Time: 20 minutes   ♣   Setting: Manual and Sauté
Pressure: High   ♣   Release: Manual

1 tablespoon oil

1 ½ pounds boneless beef, trimmed and sliced thinly (round steak or chuck roast)

¼ teaspoon black pepper

½ cup diced onion

3 cloves garlic, minced

¾ cup low-sodium beef broth

½ cup low-sodium soy sauce

2 tablespoons Truvia brown sugar blend

2 tablespoons sesame oil

¼ teaspoon red pepper flakes

1 pound broccoli, chopped

3 tablespoons water

3 tablespoons cornstarch

1. Put oil into the inner pot of the Instant Pot and select Sauté. When oil begins to sizzle, brown the beef in several small batches, taking care to brown well. After browning, remove and put into another bowl. Season with black pepper.

2. Sauté onion in pot for 2 minutes. Add garlic and sauté another minute. Add beef broth, soy sauce, brown sugar, sesame oil, and red pepper flakes. Stir to mix well.

3. Add beef and juices to mixture in inner pot. Secure lid and make sure vent is at sealing. Set on Manual at high pressure and set timer for 12 minutes.

4. After beep, turn cooker off and use quick pressure release. Remove lid.

5. In microwave bowl, steam the broccoli for 3 minutes or until desired doneness.

6. In a small bowl, stir together water and cornstarch. Add to pot and stir. Put on Sauté setting and stir some more. After mixture becomes thick, add broccoli and turn pot off.

Serving suggestion:

Serve over rice.

Exchange List Values	Basic Nutritional Values	Cholesterol 78 mg
Vegetable 1	Calories 350 (Calories from Fat 180)	Sodium 990 mg
Fat 2.0	Total Fat 20 gm	Total Carb 15 gm
Meat—medium 1.0	(Saturated Fat 6.8 gm, Polyunsat Fat 2.8 gm, Monounsat Fat 10.2 gm)	Dietary Fiber 2 gm
		Sugars 6 gm
		Protein 27 gm

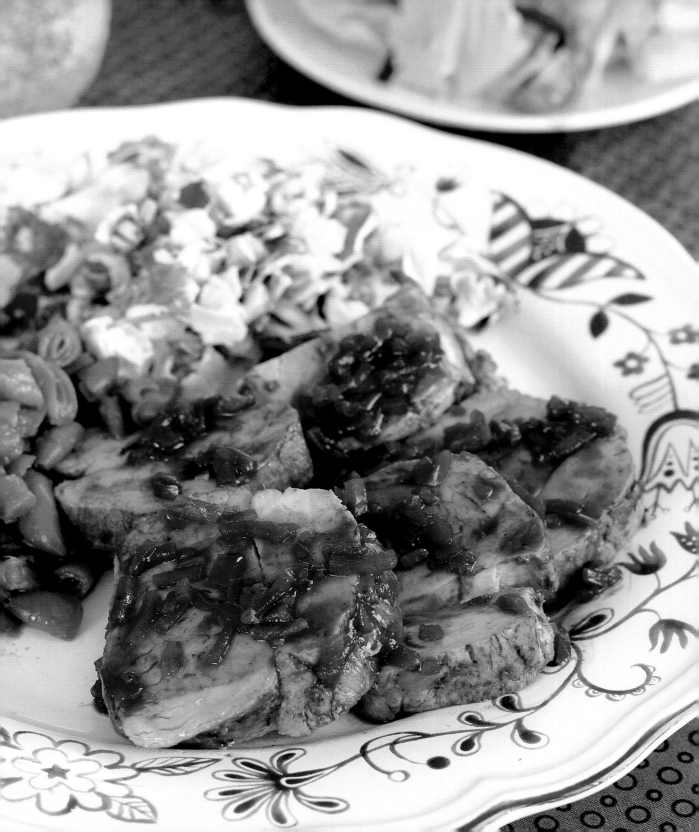

Pork Butt Roast

Marla Folkerts, Batavia, IL

Makes 6–8 servings
Prep. Time: 10 minutes 🌿 Cooking Time: 9 minutes 🌿 Setting: Manual
Pressure: High 🌿 Release: Natural

3–4-pound pork butt roast

2–3 tablespoons of your favorite rub

2 cups water

1. Place pork in the inner pot of the Instant Pot.

2. Sprinkle in the rub all over the roast and add the water, being careful not to wash off the rub.

3. Secure the lid and set the vent to sealing. Cook for 9 minutes on the Manual setting.

4. Let the pressure release naturally.

Exchange List Values

Meat—medium 8.0

Fat 0.0

Basic Nutritional Values

Calories 598 (Calories from Fat 1)

Total Fat 40 gm (Saturated Fat 15 gm, Polyunsat Fat 5.9 gm, Monounsat Fat 17.8 gm)

Cholesterol 202 mg

Sodium 152 mg

Total Carb 0 gm

Dietary Fiber 0 gm

Sugars 0 gm

Protein 57 gm

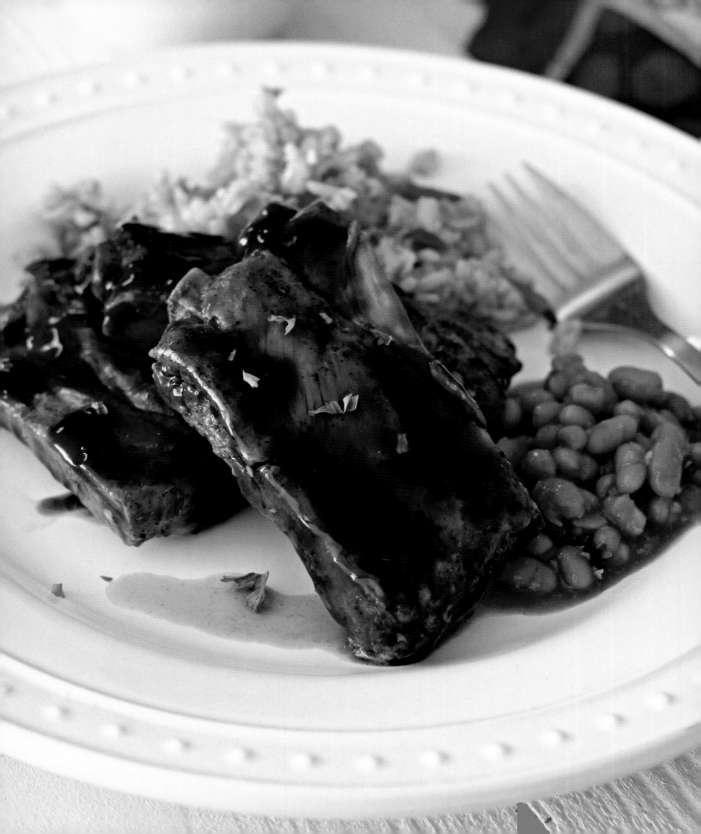

Tender Tasty Ribs

Carol Eveleth, Cheyenne, WY

Makes 2–3 servings
Prep. Time: 5 minutes & Cooking Time: 35 minutes & Setting: Manual
Pressure: High & Release: Natural

2 teaspoons salt

2 teaspoons black pepper

1 teaspoon garlic powder

1 teaspoon onion powder

1 slab baby back ribs

1 cup water

1 cup low-sugar barbecue sauce, *divided*

1. Mix salt, pepper, garlic powder, and onion powder together. Rub seasoning mixture on both sides of slab of ribs. Cut slab in half if it's too big for your Instant Pot.

2. Pour water into inner pot of the Instant Pot. Place ribs into pot, drizzle with ¼ cup of sauce, and secure lid. Make sure the vent is set to sealing.

3. Set it to Manual for 25 minutes. It will take a few minutes to heat up and seal the vent. When cook time is up, let it sit 5 minutes, then release steam by turning valve to venting. Turn oven on to broil (or heat your grill) while you're waiting for the 5-minute resting time.

4. Remove ribs from Instant Pot and place on a baking sheet. Slather on both sides with remaining ¾ cup sauce.

5. Place under broiler (or on grill) for 5–10 minutes, watching carefully so it doesn't burn. Remove and brush with a bit more sauce. Pull apart and dig in!

Exchange List Values

Meat—medium 13.5

Basic Nutritional Values

Calories 932 (Calories from Fat 405)
Total Fat 45 gm
(Saturated Fat 15.8 gm, Polyunsat Fat 7.0 gm, Monounsat Fat 19 gm)

Cholesterol 299 mg
Sodium 2570 mg
Total Carb 36 gm
Dietary Fiber 1 gm
Sugars 28 gm
Protein 96 gm

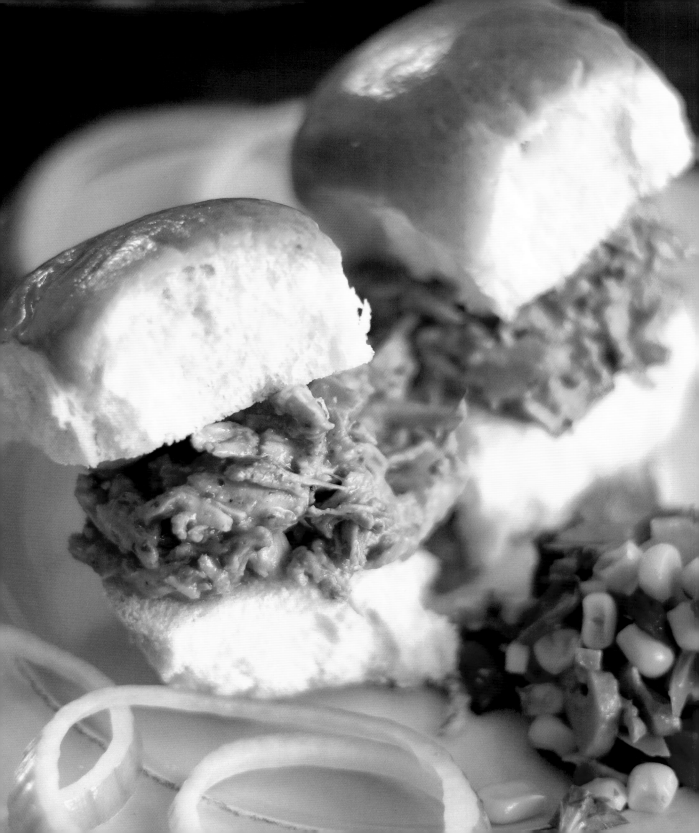

Pulled Pork

Colleen Heatwole, Burton, MI

Makes 8 servings
Prep. Time: 15 minutes   ♣   *Cooking Time: 75 minutes*   ♣   *Setting: Meat/Stew*
Pressure: High   ♣   *Release: Natural*

2 tablespoons grapeseed oil

4-pound boneless pork shoulder, cut into two pieces

2 cups low-sugar barbecue sauce, *divided*

½ cup water

1. Add oil to the inner pot of the Instant Pot and select Sauté.

2. When oil is hot, brown pork on both sides, about 3 minutes per side. Brown each half of roast separately. Remove to platter when browned.

3. Add 1 cup barbecue sauce and ½ cup water to the inner pot. Stir to combine.

4. Add browned pork and any accumulated juices to the inner pot. Secure the lid and set vent to sealing.

5. Using Meat/Stew mode, set timer to 60 minutes, on high pressure.

6. When cook time is up, allow the pressure to release naturally.

7. Carefully remove meat and shred with two forks, discarding excess fat as you shred.

8. Strain cooking liquid, reserving ½ cup. If possible use fat separator to separate fat from juices.

9. Place shredded pork in the inner pot with remaining 1 cup barbecue sauce and reserved ½ cup cooking liquid. Using Sauté function, stir to combine and bring to a simmer, stirring frequently.

Serving suggestion:

We serve on toasted buns. Our barbecue sauce of choice is Sweet Baby Ray's.

Exchange List Values

Meat—lean 7.5

Basic Nutritional Values

Calories 426 (Calories from Fat 108)
Total Fat 12 gm
(Saturated Fat 2.8 gm, Polyunsat Fat 3.5 gm, Monounsat Fat 3.9 gm)
Cholesterol 136 mg
Sodium 765 mg
Total Carb 25 gm
Dietary Fiber 1 gm
Sugars 21 gm
Protein 52 gm

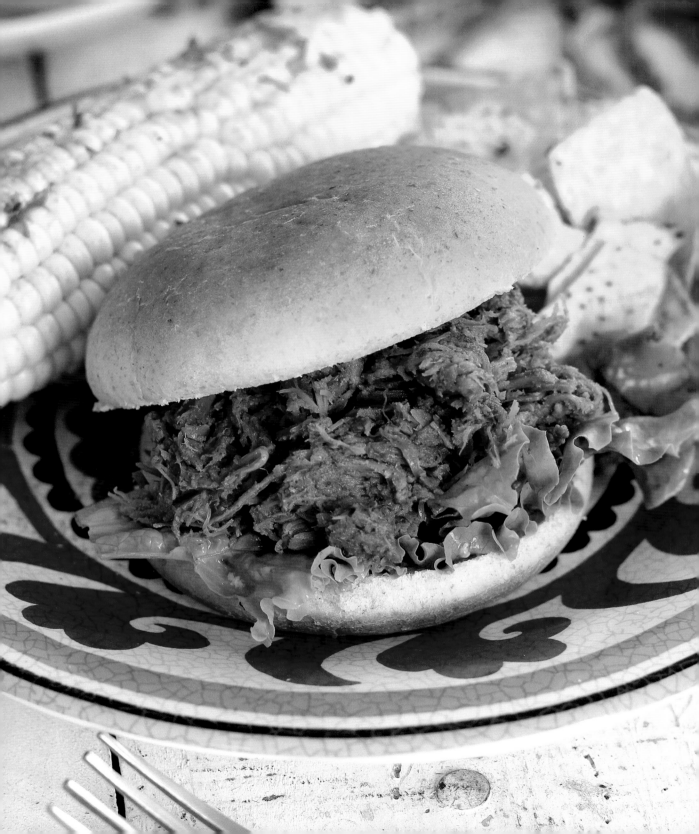

BBQ Pork Sandwiches

Carol Eveleth, Cheyenne, WY

Makes 4 servings
Prep. Time: 20 minutes   ✤   Cooking Time: 1 hour   ✤   Setting: Manual and Sauté
Pressure: High   ✤   Release: Manual

2 teaspoons salt

1 teaspoon onion powder

1 teaspoon garlic powder

2-pound pork shoulder roast, cut into 3-inch pieces

1 tablespoon olive oil

1 cup water

2 cups low-sugar barbecue sauce

1. In a small bowl, combine the salt, onion powder, and garlic powder. Season the pork with the rub.

2. Turn the Instant Pot on to Sauté. Heat the olive oil in the inner pot.

3. Add the pork to the oil and turn to coat. Add 1 cup water. Lock the lid and set vent to sealing.

4. Press Manual and cook on high pressure for 45 minutes.

5. When cooking is complete, release the pressure manually, then open the lid. Remove the pork and set on a cutting board or in a bowl. Drain the liquid from the Inner Pot.

6. Using 2 forks, shred the pork, pour barbecue sauce over the pork, then press Sauté. Simmer, 3 to 5 minutes. Press Cancel. Toss pork to mix.

Serving suggestion:
Pile the shredded BBQ pork on the bottom half of a bun. Add any additional toppings if you wish, then finish with the top half of the bun.

Exchange List Values	Basic Nutritional Values	
Meat—lean 7.5	Calories 536 (Calories from Fat 108)	Cholesterol 136 mg
		Sodium 2367 mg
	Total Fat 12 gm (Saturated Fat 3.0 gm, Polyunsat Fat 1.6 gm, Monounsat Fat 5.9 gm)	Total Carb 52 gm
		Dietary Fiber 1 gm
		Sugars 42 gm
		Protein 52 gm

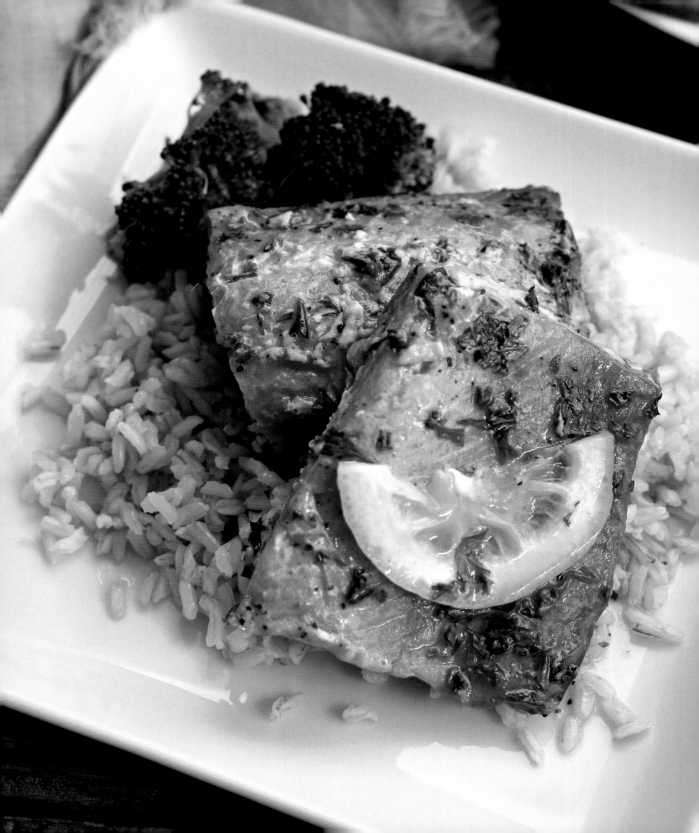

Honey Lemon Garlic Salmon

Judy Gascho, Woodburn, OR

Makes 4 servings
Prep. Time: 15 minutes & Cooking Time: 8 minutes & Setting: Manual
Pressure: High & Release: Manual

5 tablespoons olive oil

3 tablespoons agave nectar

2–3 tablespoons lemon juice

3 cloves garlic, minced

4 3–4-ounces fresh salmon fillets

Salt and pepper to taste

1–2 tablespoons minced parsley (dried or fresh)

Lemon slices, *optional*

1. Mix olive oil, agave nectar, lemon juice, and minced garlic in a bowl.

2. Place each piece of salmon on a piece of foil big enough to wrap up the piece of fish.

3. Brush each fillet generously with the olive oil mixture.

4. Sprinkle with salt, pepper, and parsley flakes.

5. Top each with a thin slice of lemon, if desired.

6. Wrap each fillet and seal well at top.

7. Place 1½ cups of water in the inner pot of your Instant Pot and place the trivet in the pot.

8. Place wrapped fillets on the trivet.

9. Close the lid and turn valve to sealing.

10. Cook on Manual at high pressure for 5–8 minutes for smaller pieces, or 10–12 minutes if they are large.

11. Carefully release pressure manually at the end of the cooking time.

12. Unwrap and enjoy.

NOTE
If you have a large fillet, you can cut it into serving pieces with your kitchen shears.

Exchange List Values

Meat—medium 3.5

Fat 1

Basic Nutritional Values

Calories 348 (Calories from Fat 198)

Total Fat 22 gm (Saturated Fat 3.6 gm, Polyunsat Fat 3.3 gm, Monounsat Fat 14 gm)

Cholesterol 57 mg

Sodium 81 mg

Total Carb 14 gm

Dietary Fiber 0 gm

Sugars 12 gm

Protein 26 gm

Side Dishes & Vegetables

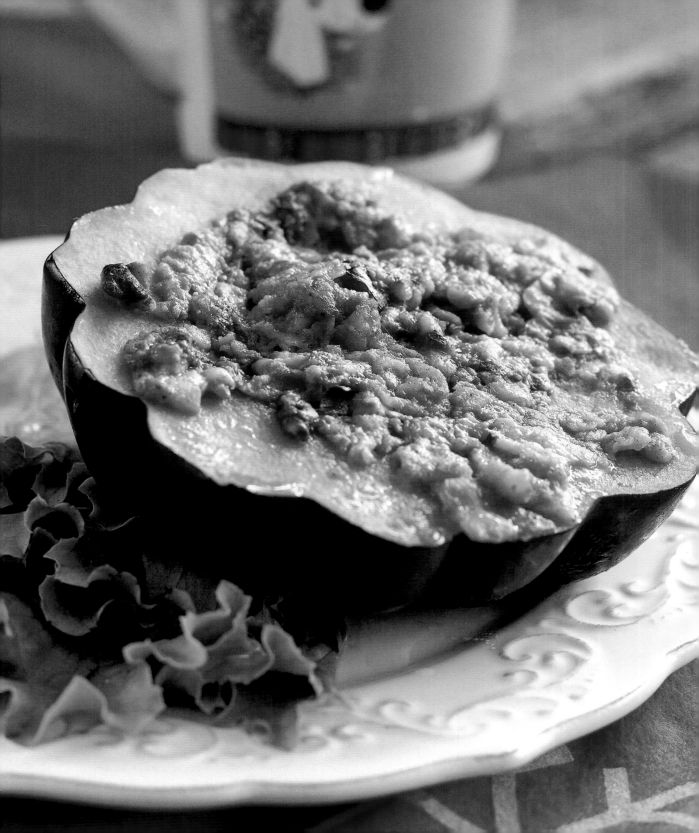

Baked Acorn Squash

Dale Peterson, Rapid City, SD

Makes 4 servings
Prep. Time: 25 minutes ⚘ Cooking Time: 5 minutes ⚘ Setting: Manual
Pressure: High ⚘ Release: Natural

2 small (1 ¼ pound each) acorn squash

½ cup cracker crumbs

¼ cup coarsely chopped pecans

2 tablespoons light, soft tub margarine, melted

2 tablespoons brown sugar

Brown sugar substitute to equal 1 tablespoon sugar

¼ teaspoon salt

¼ teaspoon ground nutmeg

2 tablespoons orange juice

1 cup water

1. Cut squash in half. Remove seeds.

2. Combine remaining ingredients. Spoon into squash halves.

3. Place the trivet inside the inner pot of the Instant Pot and pour in 1 cup water. Place the acorn squash halves on top of the trivet.

4. Secure the lid and set the vent to sealing. Press Manual and set the time for 5 minutes.

5. When cook time is up, let the pressure release naturally.

Exchange List Values

Starch 2.0
Carbohydrate 0.5
Fat 1.0

Basic Nutritional Values

Calories 229 (Calories from Fat 82)
Total Fat 9 gm
(Saturated Fat 0.8 gm, Polyunsat Fat 2.3 gm, Monounsat Fat 5.1 gm)

Cholesterol 0 mg
Sodium 314 mg
Total Carb 38 gm
Dietary Fiber 8 gm
Sugars 15 gm
Protein 3 gm

Apple Walnut Squash

Michele Ruvola, Selden, NY

Makes 4 servings
Prep. Time: 10 minutes ⚜ Cooking Time: 5 minutes ⚜ Setting: Manual
Pressure: High ⚜ Release: Natural

I cup water

2 small (1¼ pound each) acorn squash

2 tablespoons brown sugar

Brown sugar substitute to equal
1 tablespoon sugar

2 tablespoons light, soft tub margarine

3 tablespoons apple juice

1½ teaspoons ground cinnamon

¼ teaspoon salt

I cup toasted walnuts halves

I medium apple, unpeeled, chopped

1. Pour water into Instant Pot and place the trivet inside.

2. Cut squash crosswise in half. Remove seeds. Place in the Instant Pot on top of the trivet, cut sides up.

3. Combine brown sugar, brown sugar substitute, margarine, apple juice, cinnamon, and salt. Spoon into squash.

4. Secure the lid and make sure vent is set to sealing. Press Manual and set time for 5 minutes.

5. Let the pressure release naturally.

6. Combine walnuts and chopped apple. Add to center of squash when the cook time is over.

Exchange List Values	Basic Nutritional Values	
Starch 1.5	Calories 244 (Calories from Fat 96)	Cholesterol 0 mg
Fruit 1.0		Sodium 202 mg
Fat 1.5	Total Fat 11 gm (Saturated Fat 0.8 gm, Polyunsat Fat 6.5 gm, Monounsat Fat 2.4 gm)	Total Carb 39 gm
		Dietary Fiber 9 gm
		Sugars 19 gm
		Protein 4 gm

Janie's Vegetable Medley

Janie Steele, Moore, OK

Makes 8 servings
Prep Time: 25–30 minutes ⚜ Cooking Time: 4 minutes ⚜ Setting: Manual
Pressure: High ⚜ Release: Manual

Large potato, peeled and cut into small cubes

2 onions, chopped

2 carrots, sliced thin

Large green pepper, chopped

2 zucchini, chopped

8 ounces frozen green peas

¾ cup uncooked long-grain rice

2 tablespoons lemon juice

¼ cup olive oil

2 1-pound cans diced tomatoes, *divided*

I cup water, *divided*

2 tablespoons parsley, chopped

¾ teaspoon salt

I cup cheese, grated

Hot sauce, *optional*

1. Combine cubed potato, chopped onions, sliced carrots, green pepper, zucchini, peas, uncooked rice, lemon juice, olive oil, 1 can of tomatoes, and ½ cup water in the inner pot of the Instant Pot.

2. Secure the lid and make sure vent is set to sealing. Press Manual and cook for 4 minutes. Release pressure manually.

3. Remove the lid and stir in remaining ingredients except the cheese and hot sauce.

4. Serve in bowls, topped with grated cheese. Pass hot sauce to be added individually.

Exchange List Values

Starch 1.5
Vegetable 2.0
Fat 2.0

Basic Nutritional Values

Calories 260 (Calories from Fat 90)
Total Fat 10 gm
(Saturated Fat 2.5 gm, Polyunsat Fat 1.0 gm, Monounsat Fat 6.0 gm)

Cholesterol 5 mg
Sodium 580 mg
Total Carb 36 gm
Dietary Fiber 5 gm
Sugars 9 gm
Protein 9 gm

Vegetable Medley

Teena Wagner, Waterloo, ON

Makes 8 servings
Prep. Time: 20 minutes ⚜ Cooking Time: 2 minutes ⚜ Setting: Manual and Sauté
Pressure: High ⚜ Release: Manual

2 medium parsnips

4 medium carrots

1 turnip, about 4½ inches diameter

1 cup water

1 teaspoon salt

3 tablespoons sugar

2 tablespoons canola or olive oil

½ teaspoon salt

1. Clean and peel vegetables. Cut in 1-inch pieces.

2. Place the cup of water and 1 teaspoon salt into the Instant Pot's inner pot with the vegetables.

3. Secure the lid and make sure vent is set to sealing. Press Manual and set for 2 minutes.

4. When cook time is up, release the pressure manually and press Cancel. Drain the water from the inner pot.

5. Press Sauté and stir in sugar, oil, and salt. Cook until sugar is dissolved. Serve.

Exchange List Values

Starch 1.0

Basic Nutritional Values

Calories 63 (Calories from Fat 17)
Total Fat 2 gm
(Saturated Fat 0.1 gm, Polyunsat Fat 0.6 gm, Monounsat Fat 1.0 gm)

Cholesterol 0 mg
Sodium 327 mg
Total Carb 12 gm
Dietary Fiber 2 gm
Sugars 6 gm
Protein 1 gm

Best Brown Rice

Colleen Heatwhole, Burton, MI

Makes 6–12 servings
Prep. Time: 5 minutes ⚬ Cooking Time: 22 minutes ⚬ Setting: Manual
Pressure: High ⚬ Release: Natural then Manual

2 cups brown rice

2½ cups water

1. Rinse brown rice in a fine-mesh strainer.

2. Add rice and water to the inner pot of the Instant Pot.

3. Secure the lid and make sure vent is on sealing.

4. Use Manual setting and select 22 minutes cooking time on high pressure.

5. When cooking time is done, let the pressure release naturally for 10 minutes, then press Cancel and manually release any remaining pressure.

NOTE

Brown rice is my preferred rice since it is more nutritious than white rice.

I have also cooked brown rice 25 minutes and then done quick release and it worked fine.

I don't add salt until it is cooked, and how much I add if any depends on how I'm using the rice.

Exchange List Values

Carbohydrate 1.5
Fat 0.0

Basic Nutritional Values

Calories 114 (Calories from Fat 3)
Total Fat 1 gm (Saturated Fat 0.2 gm, Polyunsat Fat 0.3 gm, Monounsat Fat 0.3 gm)

Cholesterol 0 mg
Sodium 3 mg
Total Carb 23 gm
Dietary Fiber 1 gm
Sugars 0 gm
Protein 2 gm

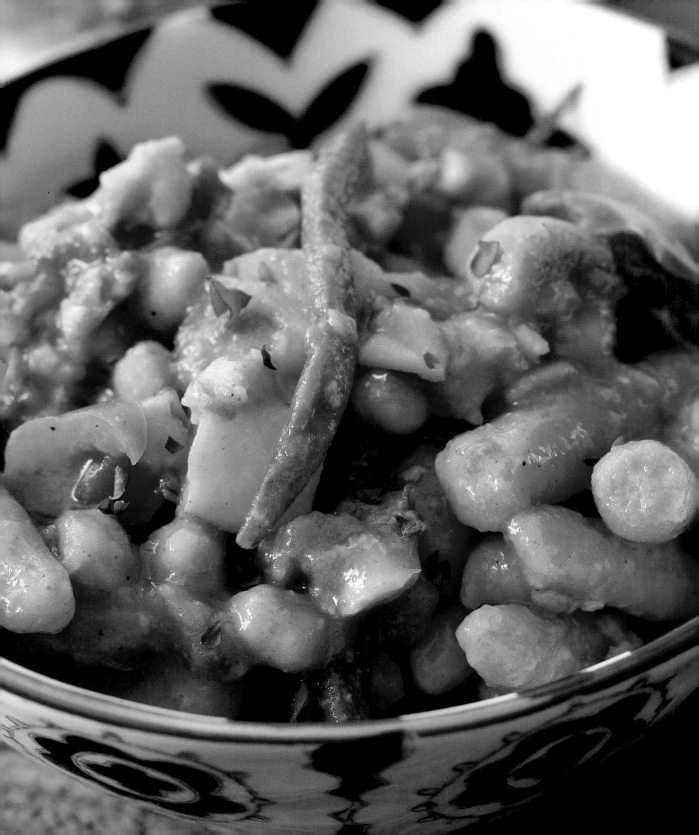

Vegetable Curry

Sheryl Shenk, Harrisonburg, VA

Makes 10 servings
Prep. Time: 25 minutes & Cooking Time: 3 minutes & Setting: Manual
Pressure: High & Release: Manual

16-ounce package baby carrots

3 medium potatoes, unpeeled, cubed

1 pound fresh or frozen green beans, cut in 2-inch pieces

1 medium green pepper, chopped

1 medium onion, chopped

1–2 cloves garlic, minced

15-ounce can garbanzo beans, drained

28-ounce can crushed tomatoes

3 teaspoons curry powder

1½ teaspoons chicken bouillon granules

1¾ cups boiling water

3 tablespoons minute tapioca

1. Combine carrots, potatoes, green beans, pepper, onion, garlic, garbanzo beans, crushed tomatoes, and curry powder in the Instant Pot.

2. Dissolve bouillon in boiling water, then stir in tapicoa. Pour over the contents of the Instant Pot and stir.

3. Secure the lid and make sure vent is set to sealing. Press Manual and set for 3 minutes.

4. When cook time is up, manually release the pressure.

Serving suggestion:
Serve over cooked brown rice.

Exchange List Values

Starch 1.0
Vegetable 3.0

Basic Nutritional Values

Calories 166 (Calories from Fat 10)
Total Fat 1 gm
(Saturated Fat 0.1 gm, Polyunsat Fat 0.5 gm, Monounsat Fat 0.2 gm)
Cholesterol 0 mg
Sodium 436 mg
Total Carb 35 gm
Dietary Fiber 8 gm
Sugars 10 gm
Protein 6 gm

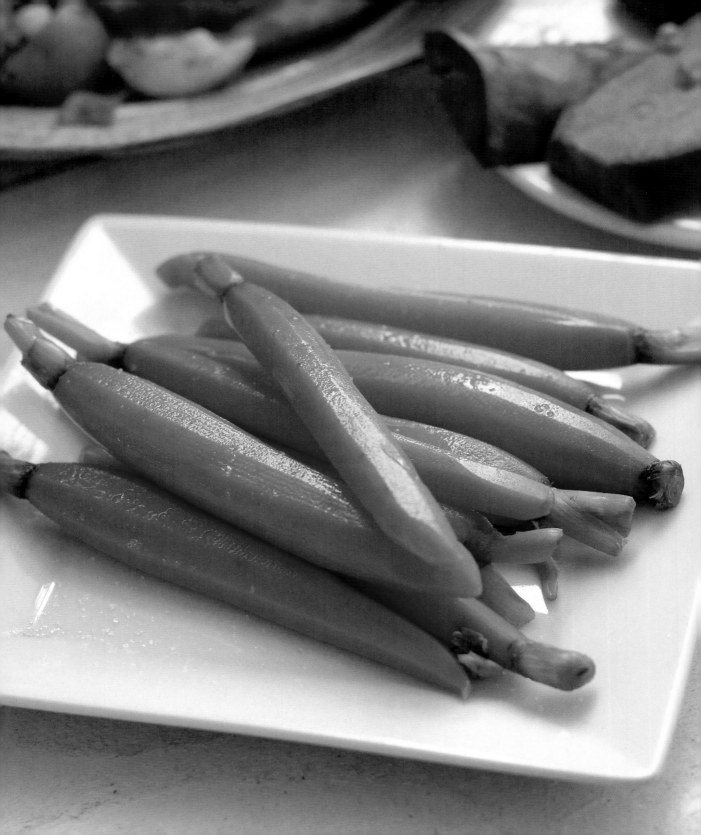

Simple Salted Carrots

Hope Comerford
Clinton Township, MI

Makes 4 servings
Prep Time: 5 minutes   ⚜   Cooking Time: 2 minutes   ⚜   Setting: Manual then Sauté
Pressure: High   ⚜   Release: Manual

1 pound package baby carrots
1 cup water
1 tablespoon margarine
sea salt to taste

1. Combine the carrots and water in the inner pot of the Instant Pot.

2. Seal the lid and make sure the vent is on sealing. Select Manual for 2 minutes.

3. When cooking time is done, release the pressure manually, then pour the carrots into a strainer.

4. Wipe the inner pot dry. Select the Sauté function and add the margarine.

5. When the margarine is melted, add the carrots back into the inner pot and sauté them until they are coated well with the margarine.

6. Remove the carrots and sprinkle them with the sea salt to taste before serving.

Exchange List Values

Vegetable 2.0
Fat 0.5

Basic Nutritional Values

Calories 262 (Calories from Fat 1)
Total Fat 3 gm
(Saturated Fat 1.1 gm, Polyunsat Fat 0.6 gm, Monounsat Fat 1.2 gm)
Cholesterol 124 mg
Sodium 75 mg
Total Carb 50 gm
Dietary Fiber 0 gm
Sugars 28 gm
Protein 6 gm

Corn on the Cob

Hope Comerford, Clinton Township, MI

Makes 6 servings
Prep. Time: 10 minutes & Cooking Time: 2 minutes & Setting: Manual
Pressure: High & Release: Manual

1 cup water

6 small ears of corn, husked and ends cut off

1. Place the trivet in the bottom of the Instant Pot and pour in the water.

2. Place the ears of corn inside.

3. Seal the lid and make sure vent is set to sealing. Press Manual and set time for 2 minutes.

4. When cook time is up, release the pressure manually.

Exchange List Values

Starch 1.0

Basic Nutritional Values

Calories 68 (Calories from Fat 5)
Total Fat 1 gm (Saturated Fat 0.1 gm, Polyunsat Fat 0.3 gm, Monounsat Fat 0.2 gm)
Cholesterol 0 mg
Sodium 3 mg
Total Carb 16 gm
Dietary Fiber 2 gm
Sugars 2 gm
Protein 2 gm

Caramelized Onions

Mrs. J.E. Barthold, Bethlehem, PA

Makes 8 servings
Prep. Time: 10 minutes ✤ Cooking Time: 35 minutes ✤ Setting: Sauté and Manual
Pressure: High ✤ Release: Manual

4 tablespoons margarine

6 large Vidalia or other sweet onions, sliced into thin half rings

10-ounce can chicken, or vegetable, broth

1. Press Sauté on the Instant Pot. Add in the margarine and let melt.

2. Once the margarine is melted, stir in the onions and sauté for about 5 minutes. Pour in the broth and then press Cancel.

3. Secure the lid and make sure vent is set to sealing. Press Manual and set time for 20 minutes.

4. When cook time is up, release the pressure manually. Remove the lid and press Sauté. Stir the onion mixture for about 10 more minutes, allowing extra liquid to cook off.

Serving Suggestion:

Serve as a side dish, or use onions and liquid to flavor soups or stews, or as topping for pizza.

Exchange List Values

Vegetable 3.0
Fat 1.0

Basic Nutritional Values

Calories 123 (Calories from Fat 57)
Total Fat 6 gm
(Saturated Fat 1.1 gm, Polyunsat Fat 2.0 gm, Monounsat Fat 2.7 gm)

Cholesterol 1 mg
Sodium 325 mg
Total Carb 15 gm
Dietary Fiber 3 gm
Sugars 11 gm
Protein 2 gm

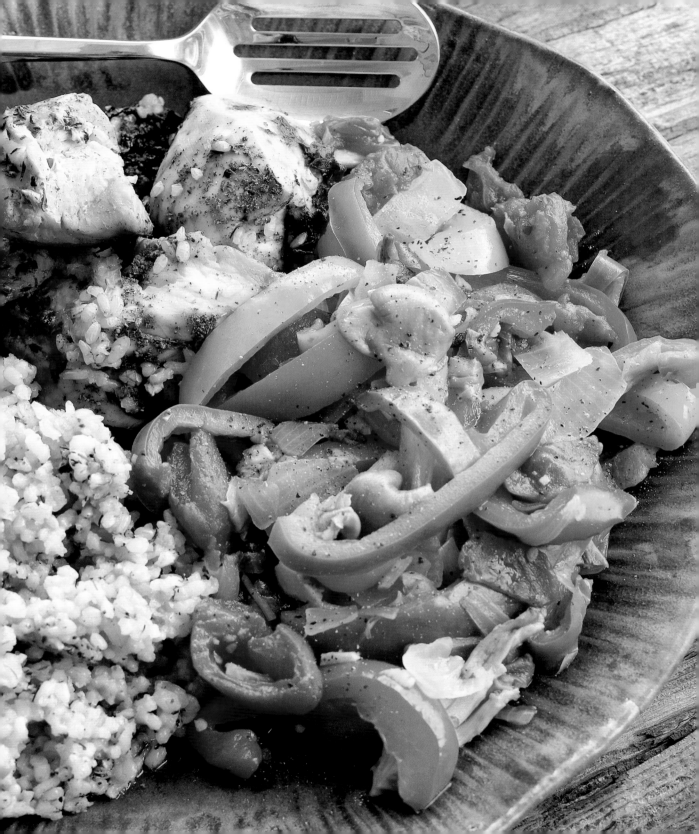

Italian Wild Mushrooms

Connie Johnson, Loudon, NH

Makes 10 servings
Prep. Time: 30 minutes ⚜ Cooking Time: 3 minutes ⚜ Setting: Sauté and Manual
Pressure: High ⚜ Release: Manual

2 tablespoons canola oil

2 large onions, chopped

4 garlic cloves, minced

3 large red bell peppers, chopped

3 large green bell peppers, chopped

12-ounce package oyster mushrooms, cleaned and chopped

3 fresh bay leaves

10 fresh basil leaves, chopped

1 teaspoon salt

1½ teaspoons pepper

28-ounce can Italian plum tomatoes, crushed or chopped

1. Press Sauté on the Instant Pot and add in the oil. Once the oil is heated, add the onions, garlic, peppers, and mushroom to the oil. Sauté just until mushrooms begin to turn brown.

2. Add remaining ingredients. Stir well.

3. Secure the lid and make sure vent is set to sealing. Press Manual and set time for 3 minutes.

4. When cook time is up, release the pressure manually. Discard bay leaves.

Serving Suggestion:
Good as an appetizer or on pita bread, or serve over rice or pasta for main dish.

Exchange List Values

Vegetable 3.0
Fat 0.5

Basic Nutritional Values

Calories 82 (Calories from Fat 29)
Total Fat 3 gm
(Saturated Fat 0.2 gm, Polyunsat Fat 1.0 gm, Monounsat Fat 1.7 gm)

Cholesterol 0 mg
Sodium 356 mg
Total Carb 13 gm
Dietary Fiber 4 gm
Sugars 8 gm
Protein 3 gm

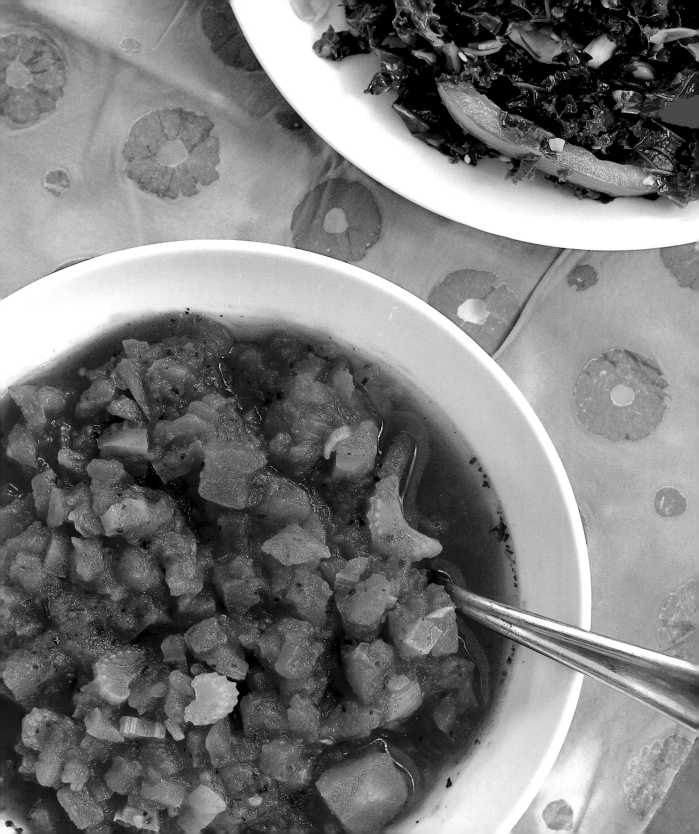

Stewed Tomatoes

Michelle Showalter, Bridgewater, VA

Makes 12 servings
Prep. Time: 10 minutes ⚜ *Cooking Time: 25 minutes* ⚜ *Setting: Manual*
Pressure: High ⚜ *Release: Manual* ⚜ *Oven Time: 8–10 minutes*

2 quarts canned tomatoes

½ cup water

2½ tablespoons sugar

Sugar substitute to equal
1½ tablespoons sugar

½ teaspoons salt

Dash of pepper

2 cups bread cubes

1½ tablespoons light, soft tub
margarine

1. Place tomatoes in Instant Pot along with the water and sprinkle with sugar, sugar substitute, salt, and pepper.

2. Secure the lid and make sure the vent is set to sealing. Press Manual and set the time for 15 minutes.

3. When cook time is up, release the pressure manually.

4. Pour tomatoes into a baking dish.

5. Lightly toast bread cubes in melted margarine. Spread over tomatoes.

6. Bake in oven at 400 degrees for 8–10 minutes.

Exchange List Values

Vegetable 2.0

Basic Nutritional Values

Calories 62 (Calories from Fat 9)
Total Fat 1 gm
(Saturated Fat 0.0 gm, Polyunsat Fat 0.4 gm, Monounsat Fat 0.4 gm)

Cholesterol 0 mg
Sodium 377 mg
Total Carb 13 gm
Dietary Fiber 2 gm
Sugars 7 gm
Protein 2 gm

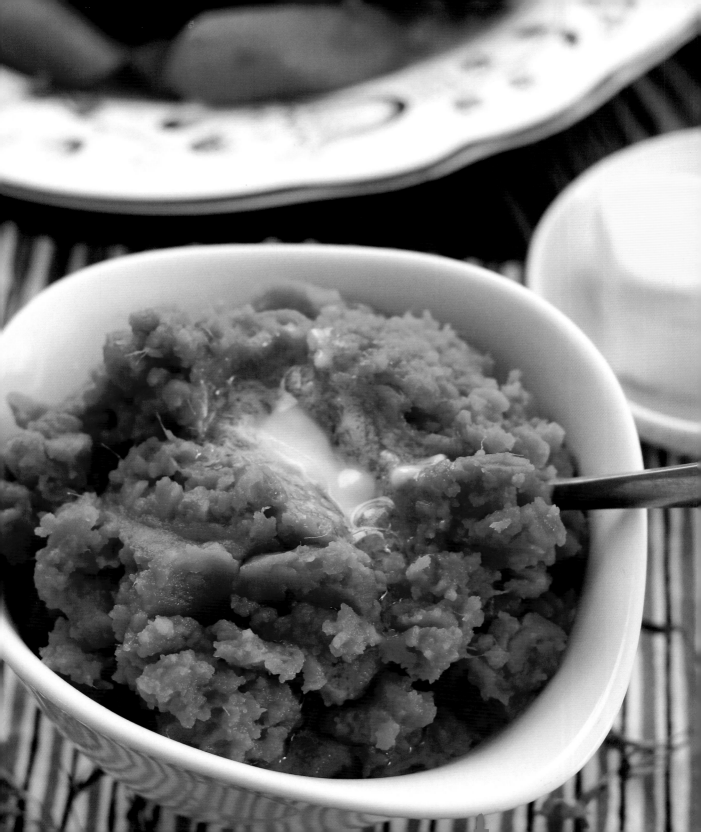

Sweet Potato Puree

Colleen Heatwole, Burton, MI

Makes 4 servings
Prep. Time: 10 minutes ⚭ Cooking Time: 6 minutes ⚭ Setting: Manual
Pressure: High ⚭ Release: Manual

3 pounds sweet potatoes, peeled and cut into roughly 2-inch cubes

1 cup water

2 tablespoons margarine

1 teaspoon salt

1 teaspoon brown sugar substitute such as Truvia

2 teaspoons lemon juice

½ teaspoon cinnamon

⅛ teaspoon nutmeg, *optional*

1. Place sweet potatoes and water in inner pot of the Instant Pot.

2. Secure the lid, make sure vent is at sealing, then cook for 6 minutes on high using the Manual setting.

3. Manually release the pressure when cook time is up.

4. Drain sweet potatoes and place in large mixing bowl. Mash with potato masher or hand mixer.

5. Once thoroughly mashed, add remaining ingredients.

6. Taste and adjust seasonings to taste.

7. Serve immediately while still hot.

Exchange List Values

Carbohydrate 4.0
Fat 1

Basic Nutritional Values

Calories 352 (Calories from Fat 54)
Total Fat 6 gm (Saturated Fat 1.1 gm, Polyunsat Fat 1.8 gm, Monounsat Fat 2.7 gm)

Cholesterol 0 mg
Sodium 735 mg
Total Carb 70 gm
Dietary Fiber 10 gm
Sugars 16 gm
Protein 5 gm

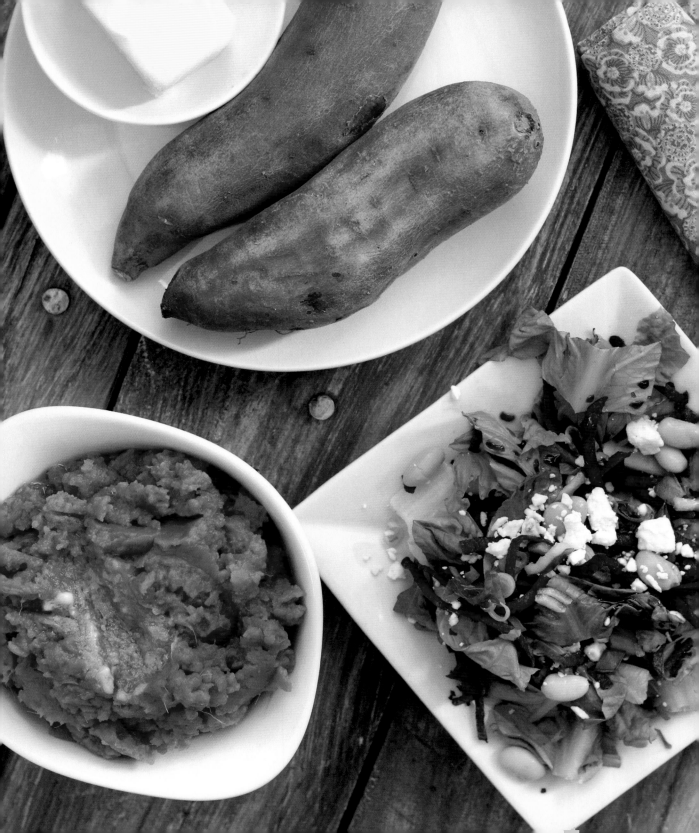

Perfect Sweet Potatoes

Brittney Horst, Lititz, PA

Makes 4–6 servings
Prep. Time: 5 minutes ⚹ Cooking Time: 15 minutes ⚹ Setting: Manual
Pressure: High ⚹ Release: Natural

4–6 medium sweet potatoes
1 cup of water

1. Scrub skin of sweet potatoes with a brush until clean. Pour water into inner pot of the Instant Pot. Place steamer basket in the bottom of the inner pot. Place sweet potatoes on top of steamer basket.

2. Secure the lid and turn valve to seal.

3. Select the Manual mode and set to pressure cook on high for 15 minutes.

4. Allow pressure to release naturally (about 10 minutes).

5. Once the pressure valve lowers, remove lid and serve immediately.

NOTE
You can store cooked sweet potatoes in the fridge for 3–4 days in an airtight container.

TIP
Super large sweet potatoes need more than 15 minutes! I tried one mega sweet potato and it was not cooked in the center. Maybe 20 minutes will do.

Exchange List Values

Carbohydrate 2
Fat 0.0

Basic Nutritional Values

Calories 112 (Calories from Fat 1)
Total Fat 0 gm
(Saturated Fat 0 gm, Polyunsat Fat 0.0 gm, Monounsat Fat 0 gm)

Cholesterol 0 mg
Sodium 72 mg
Total Carb 26 gm
Dietary Fiber 4 gm
Sugars 5 gm
Protein 2 gm

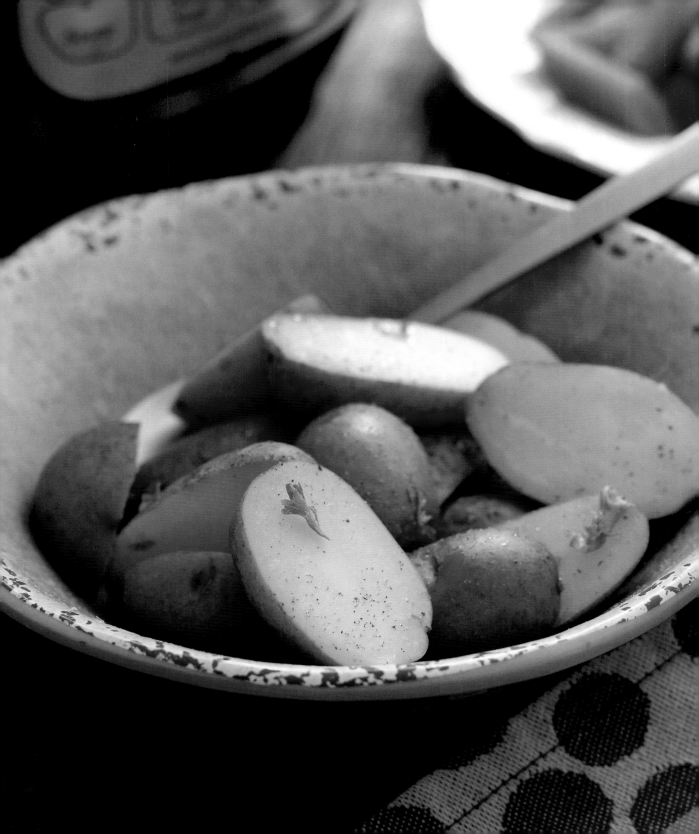

Potatoes with Parsley

Colleen Heatwole, Burton, MI

Makes 4 servings
Prep. Time: 10 minutes ☙ Cooking Time: 5 minutes ☙ Setting: Sauté then Manual
Pressure: High ☙ Release: Manual

3 tablespoons margarine, *divided*

2 pounds medium red potatoes (about 2 ounces each), halved lengthwise

1 clove garlic, minced

½ teaspoon salt

½ cup low-sodium chicken broth

2 tablespoons chopped fresh parsley

1. Place 1 tablespoon margarine in the inner pot of the Instant Pot and select Sauté.

2. After margarine is melted, add potatoes, garlic, and salt, stirring well.

3. Sauté 4 minutes, stirring frequently.

4. Add chicken broth and stir well.

5. Seal lid, make sure vent is on sealing, then select Manual for 5 minutes on high pressure.

6. When cooking time is up, manually release the pressure.

7. Strain potatoes, toss with remaining 2 tablespoons margarine and chopped parsley, and serve immediately.

Exchange List Values

Carbohydrate 2.5
Fat 2

Basic Nutritional Values

Calories 237 (Calories from Fat 1)
Total Fat 9 gm
(Saturated Fat 17 gm, Polyunsat Fat 2.7 gm, Monounsat Fat 4.1 gm)
Cholesterol 0 mg
Sodium 389 mg
Total Carb 37 gm
Dietary Fiber 4 gm
Sugars 3 gm
Protein 5 gm

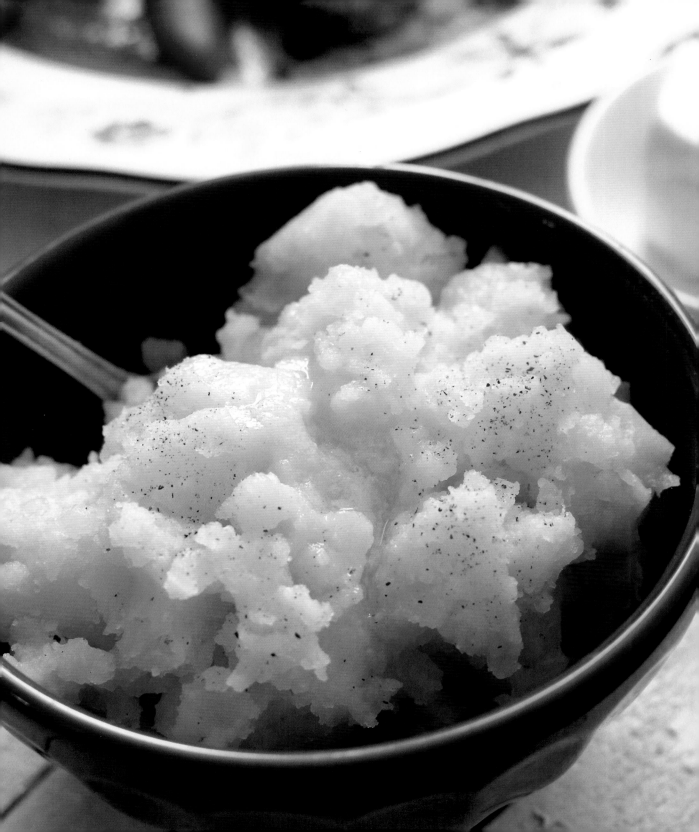

Mashed Potatoes

Colleen Heatwole, Burton, MI

Makes 3–4 servings
Prep. Time: 10 minutes ⚭ Cooking Time: 5 minutes ⚭ Setting: Manual
Pressure: High ⚭ Release: Manual

1 cup water

6 medium size potatoes, peeled and quartered

2 tablespoons margarine

½ to ¾ cup skim milk, warmed

Salt and pepper to taste

1. Add 1 cup water to the inner pot of the Instant Pot. Put the steamer basket in the pot and place potatoes in the basket.

2. Seal the lid and make sure vent is at sealing. Using Manual mode, select 5 minutes cook time, high pressure.

3. When cook time ends, do a manual release. Use a fork to test potatoes. If needed, relock lid and cook at high pressure a few minutes more.

4. Transfer potatoes to large mixing bowl. Mash using hand mixer, stirring in margarine. Gradually add warmed milk. Season with salt and pepper to taste.

NOTE

A few lumps are okay . . . that lets you know they are real potatoes. Some people prefer a ricer to a hand mixer for perfect, lump-free mashed potatoes. I used to do it that way, but my family is fine with hand mixer mashed potatoes.

Exchange List Values

Starch 2.0

Fat 0.5

Basic Nutritional Values

Calories 222 (Calories from Fat 54)

Total Fat 6 gm (Saturated Fat 1.6 gm, Polyunsat Fat 1.8 gm, Monounsat Fat 2.7 gm)

Cholesterol 1 mg

Sodium 122 mg

Total Carb 40 gm

Dietary Fiber 5 gm

Sugars 5 gm

Protein 5 gm

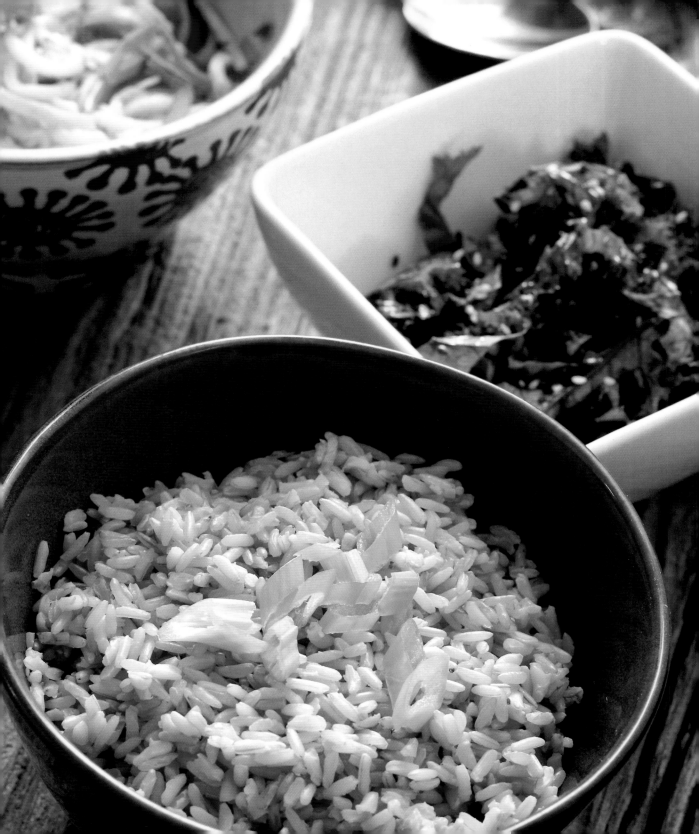

Brown Rice

Marla Folkerts, Batavia, IL

Makes 7 servings
Prep. Time: 4–5 minutes ⚜ Cooking Time: 22–25 minutes ⚜ Setting: Sauté then Manual
Pressure: High ⚜ Release: Natural

½ cup finely diced onion

2 tablespoons butter

1½ cups brown rice

1¾ cups low-sodium chicken broth

1. Use the Sauté function on the Instant Pot to sauté the diced onion and butter in the inner pot.

2. When the onions are translucent, place rice and broth in the inner pot.

3. Secure the lid, make sure the vent is at sealing, then use the Manual setting for 22–25 minutes on high pressure.

4. Let the pressure release naturally, then fluff!

Exchange List Values

Starch 2.0

Fat 1.0

Basic Nutritional Values

Calories 182 (Calories from Fat 45)

Total Fat 5 gm (Saturated Fat 2.3 gm, Polyunsat Fat 0.5 gm, Monounsat Fat 1.4 gm)

Cholesterol 9 mg

Sodium 17 mg

Total Carb 31 gm

Dietary Fiber 1.2 gm

Sugars 1 gm

Protein 3 gm

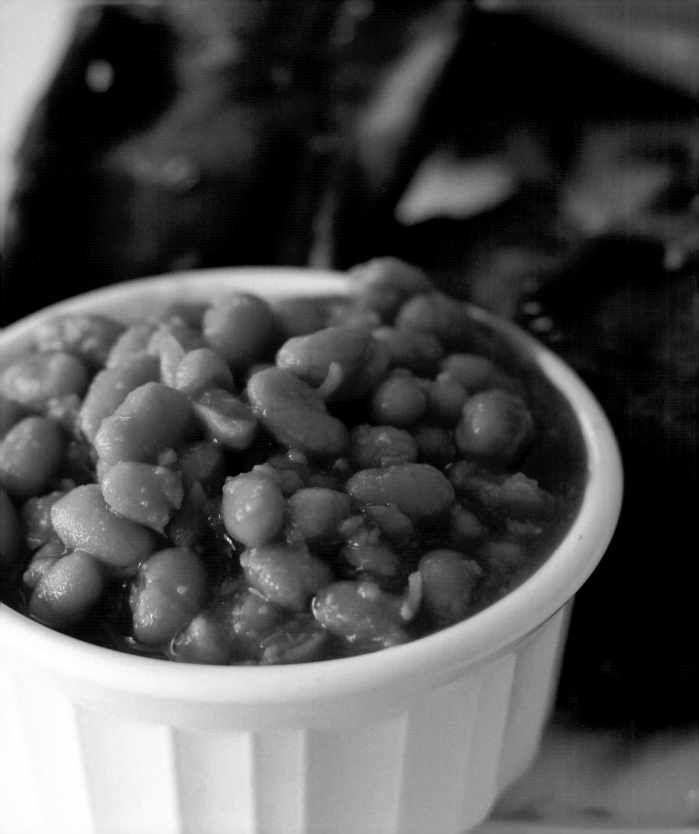

Baked Pinto Beans

Janie Steele, Moore, OK

Makes 8 servings
Prep. Time: 15 minutes   ⚜   *Cooking Time: 1 hour 30 minutes*   ⚜   *Setting: Bean/Chili and Sauté*
Pressure: High   ⚜   *Release: Natural*

1 pound dry pinto beans

1 tablespoon sea salt

6 cups water

6 slices bacon, diced

1 onion, diced

¾ cup molasses

¼ cup brown sugar substitute such as Truvia brown sugar blend

1½ teaspoons dry mustard

¾ cup low-sugar ketchup

½ teaspoon salt

½ teaspoon garlic

1½ teaspoons white wine vinegar

½ teaspoon chili powder

½ teaspoon Worcestershire sauce

1. Put beans, salt, and water in the inner pot of the Instant Pot.

2. Secure the lid and make sure vent is at sealing. Press the Bean/Chili setting and set on normal for 1 hour.

3. Let the pressure release naturally, then drain the beans. Remove the beans from the pot and set aside.

4. Sauté the bacon and onion in inner pot until the bacon is crisp and onion is translucent.

5. Mix seasonings in a bowl

6. Return beans to pot; stir.

7. Pour seasonings over beans, then stir.

8. Secure the lid and make sure vent is at sealing. Press the Bean/Chili setting and set for 30 minutes.

9. Let pressure release naturally then remove lid. Let sit to thicken.

Exchange List Values

Protein 0.5
Starch 3.0
Fat 0.0

Basic Nutritional Values

Calories 243 (Calories from Fat 27)
Total Fat 3 gm
(Saturated Fat 0.9 gm, Polyunsat Fat 0.4 gm, Monounsat Fat 1.2 gm)

Cholesterol 7 mg
Sodium 605 mg
Total Carb 48 gm
Dietary Fiber 3 gm
Sugars 37 gm
Protein 7 gm

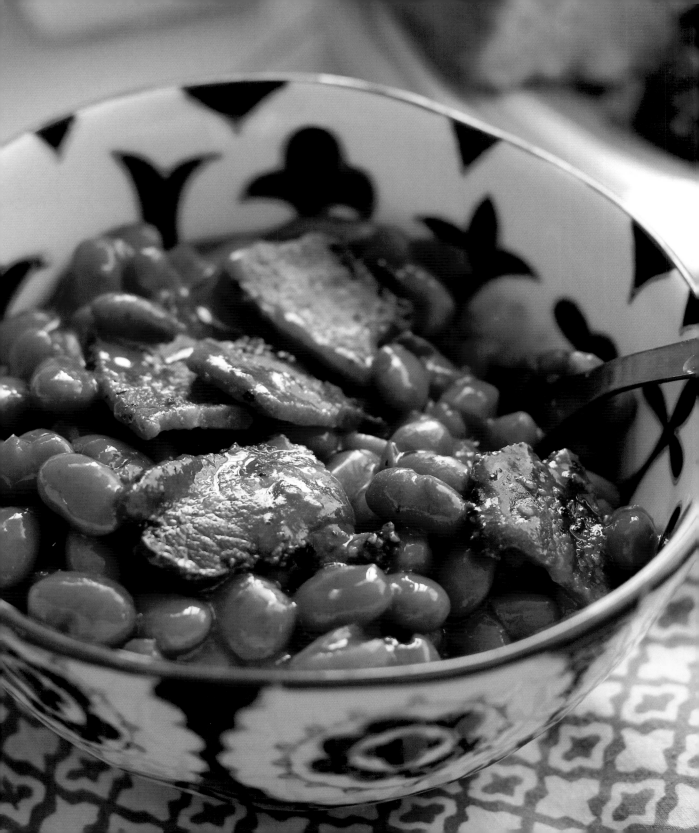

Baked Navy Beans

Colleen Heatwole, Burton, MI

Makes 8 servings
Prep. Time: 15 minutes ⚜ *Cooking Time: 25 minutes* ⚜ *Setting: Manual then Slow Cook*
Pressure: High ⚜ *Release: Natural then Manual*

I pound navy beans, cleaned, rinsed, soaked overnight in 8 cups water mixed with I tablespoon salt

10 ounces (about 8 slices) thick sliced bacon, cut into ½-inch pieces

I large onion, chopped

2½ cups water

½ cup molasses

½ cup low-sugar ketchup

2 tablespoons Truvia brown sugar blend

I teaspoon dry mustard

½ teaspoon salt

¼ teaspoon ground black pepper

1. Using Sauté function, cook bacon in the inner pot of the Instant Pot until crisp, about 5 minutes, stirring frequently.

2. Remove bacon using slotted spoon and place on plate lined with paper towels.

3. Cook the onion in bacon fat left in the inner pot until tender, about 3 minutes, stirring frequently and scraping up the brown bits on the bottom of the pot as the onion cooks.

4. Add water, molasses, ketchup, brown sugar, dry mustard, salt, and pepper and stir to combine. Stir in the soaked beans.

5. Secure lid and make sure vent is on sealing. Select Manual at high pressure and set for 25 minutes cook time.

6. When timer on pot beeps, let pressure release naturally for 10 minutes, then do a quick release for the remaining pressure.

7. Discard any beans floating on top. Check beans for tenderness. If not done, pressure-cook a few minutes longer.

8. Stir in cooked bacon. Using Slow Cook function, cook beans uncovered until sauce is desired consistency. Stir frequently to avoid burning the sauce.

NOTE

Beans vary in length of time needed to cook depending on age and variety. Soaked beans cook faster and have a slightly more desirable consistency after cooking.

Exchange List Values

Protein 0.5
Starch 2.5
Fat 0.0

Basic Nutritional Values

Calories 201 (Calories from Fat 12)
Total Fat 4 gm (Saturated Fat 1.2 gm, Polyunsat Fat 0.5 gm, Monounsat Fat 1.6 gm)

Cholesterol 9 mg
Sodium 572 mg
Total Carb 35 gm
Dietary Fiber 3 gm
Sugars 22 gm
Protein 7 gm

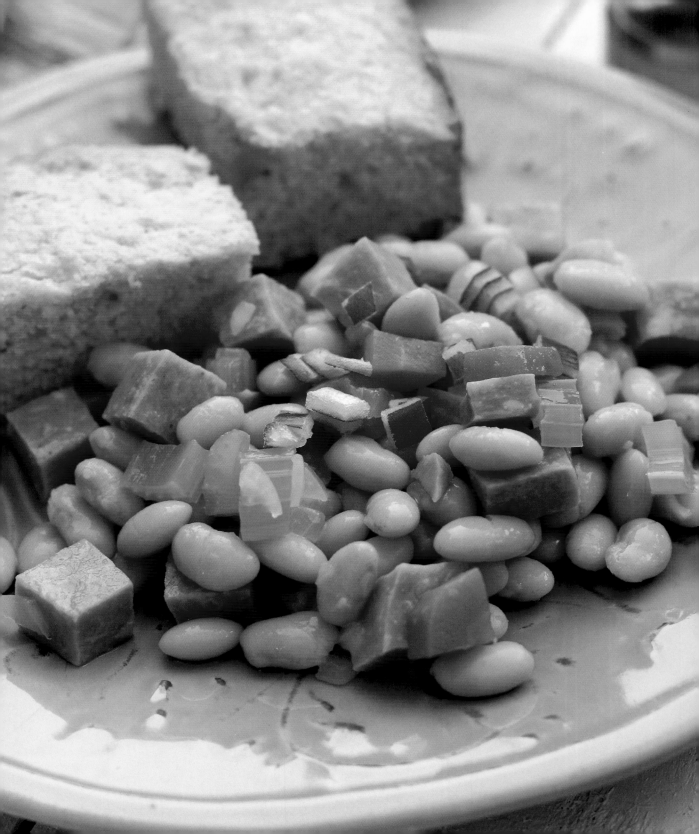

Old Fashioned Ham 'n' Beans

Carolyn Spohn, Shawnee, KS

Makes 8 servings
Prep. Time: 20 minutes ⚹ Cooking Time: 30–35 minutes ⚹ Setting: Meat or Soup/Stew
Pressure: High ⚹ Release: Natural or Manual

Meaty ham bone (with as much fat removed as possible) or 2–3 ham hocks

2 cups great northern beans, sorted and rinsed

2 medium carrots, chopped

1 medium onion, chopped

2 stalks celery, chopped

2 cloves garlic, sliced or minced

4–6 cups broth or water (depending on how "brothy" you want your beans)

Finely chopped onion for garnish, *optional*

1. Place all ingredients in the inner pot of the Instant Pot, except for finely chopped onion. Seal the lid, make sure vent is at sealing, and cook on either the Meat or Stew/Soup setting for 30 to 35 minutes.

2. Release pressure manually or let it release naturally.

3. Check beans to be sure they are fully cooked. If necessary, pressure cook a while longer, and release pressure the same as in step 2.

4. Remove ham bone or hocks and trim off the skin, bone, gristle and visible fat. Return meat to cooker and leave on Keep Warm setting.

5. Serve with chopped onion as a garnish if desired.

Serving suggestion:

Very good with cornbread.

Exchange List Values

Starch 1.5
Meat—lean 4.5
Other
   Carbohydrate 0.5

Basic Nutritional Values

Calories 374 (Calories from Fat 99)
Total Fat 11 gm
   (Saturated Fat 3.5 gm, Polyunsat Fat 1.7 gm, Monounsat Fat 4.5 gm)

Cholesterol 70 mg
Sodium 849 mg
Total Carb 32 gm
Dietary Fiber 8 gm
Sugars 2 gm
Protein 36 gm

Desserts

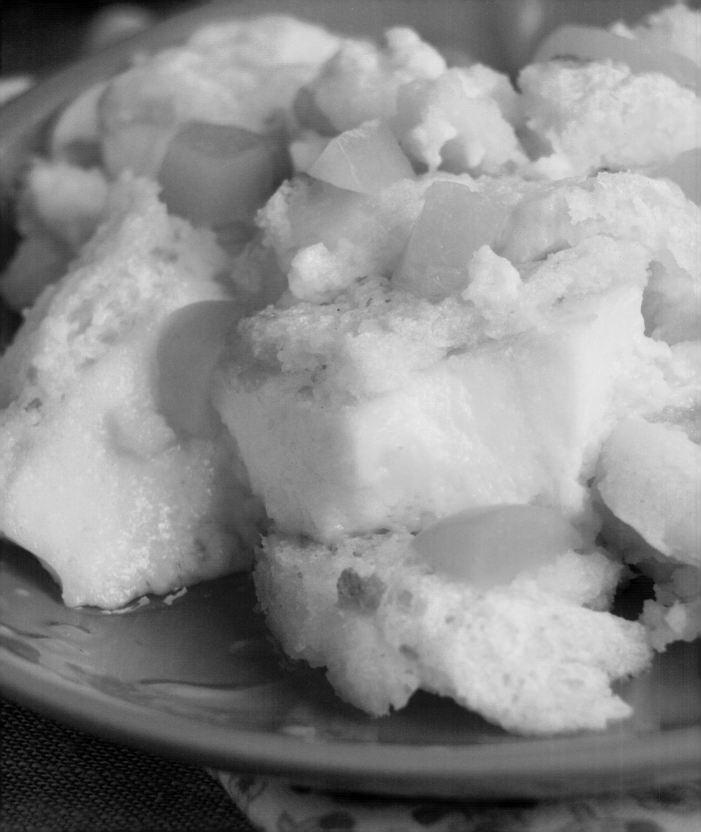

Lemon Pudding Cake

Jean Butzer, Batavia, NY

Makes 6 servings
Prep. Time: 15 minutes ⚜ Cooking Time: 50 minutes ⚜ Setting: Steam
Release: Manual ⚜ Cooling Time: 2–4 hours

3 eggs, separated

1 teaspoon grated lemon peel

¼ cup lemon juice

1 tablespoon melted light, soft tub margarine

1½ cups fat-free half-and-half

½ cup sugar

Sugar substitute to equal 2 tablespoons sugar

¼ cup flour

⅛ teaspoon salt

1 cup water

1. Beat egg whites until stiff peaks form. Set aside.

2. Beat egg yolks. Blend in lemon peel, lemon juice, margarine, and half-and-half.

3. In separate bowl, combine sugar, sugar substitute, flour, and salt. Add to egg-lemon mixture, beating until smooth.

4. Fold into beaten egg whites.

5. Spoon into a greased and floured 7" springform pan. Cover with foil.

6. Place the trivet into your Instant Pot with 1 cup of water. Place a foil sling on top of the trivet, then place the springform pan on top of the trivet.

7. Secure the lid and make sure lid is set to sealing. Press Manual and set time for 40 minutes.

8. Perform a quick release of the pressure when cooking time is done. Remove the springform pan carefully using hot pads with the foil sling and let cool on a cooling rack.

Exchange List Values

Carbohydrate 2.0

Fat 0.5

Basic Nutritional Values

Calories 169 (Calories from Fat 37)

Total Fat 4 gm (Saturated Fat 1.5 gm, Polyunsat Fat 0.5 gm, Monounsat Fat 1.4 gm)

Cholesterol 111 mg

Sodium 185 mg

Total Carb 27 gm

Dietary Fiber 0 gm

Sugars 20 gm

Protein 5 gm

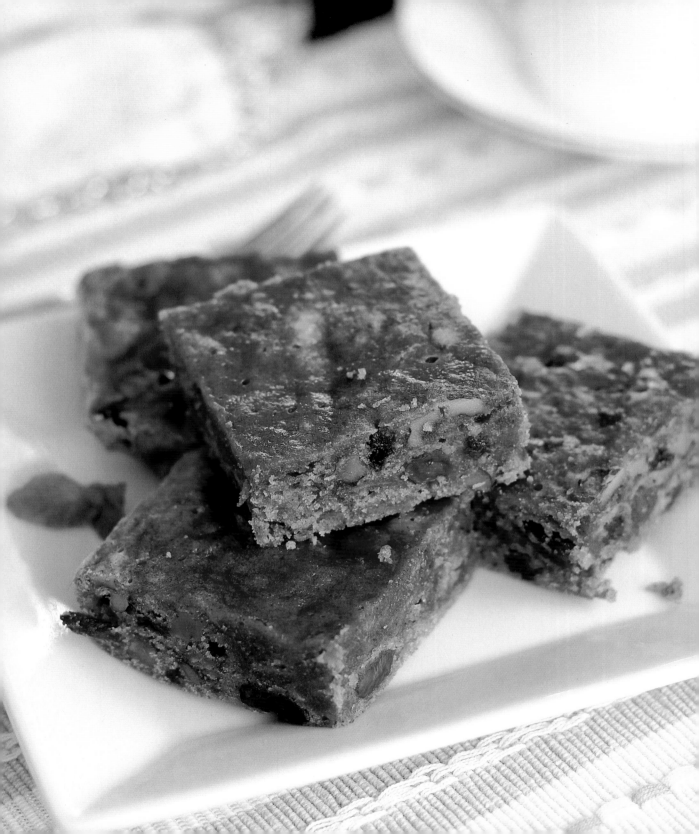

Carrot Cake

Colleen Heatwole, Burton, MI

Makes 10 servings
Prep. Time: 35 minutes ⚜ Cooking Time: 50 minutes ⚜ Setting: Steam
Release: Manual ⚜ Cooling Time: 2–4 hours

⅓ cup canola oil

2 eggs

1 tablespoon hot water

½ cup grated raw carrots

¾ cup flour and 2 tablespoons flour, *divided*

¾ cup sugar

½ teaspoon baking powder

⅛ teaspoon salt

¼ teaspoon ground allspice

½ teaspoon ground cinnamon

⅛ teaspoon ground cloves

½ cup chopped nuts

½ cup raisins or chopped dates

1 cup water

1. In large bowl, beat oil, eggs, and water for 1 minute.

2. Add carrots. Mix well.

3. Stir together flour, sugar, baking powder, salt, allspice, cinnamon, and cloves. Add to creamed mixture.

4. Toss nuts and raisins in bowl with 2 tablespoons flour. Add to creamed mixture. Mix well.

5. Pour into greased and floured 7" springform pan and cover with foil.

6. Place the trivet into your Instant Pot and pour in 1 cup of water. Place a foil sling on top of the trivet, then place the springform pan on top.

7. Secure the lid and make sure lid is set to sealing. Press Steam and set for 50 minutes.

8. When cook time is up, release the pressure manually, then carefully remove the springform pan by using hot pads to lift the pan up by the foil sling. Place on a cooling rack until cool.

Exchange List Values

Carbohydrate 2.0
Fat 3.0

Basic Nutritional Values

Calories 274 (Calories from Fat 147)
Total Fat 16 gm
    (Saturated Fat 1.5 gm, Polyunsat Fat 6.4 gm, Monounsat Fat 7.6 gm)

Cholesterol 43 mg
Sodium 66 mg
Total Carb 30 gm
Dietary Fiber 1 gm
Sugars 20 gm
Protein 4 gm

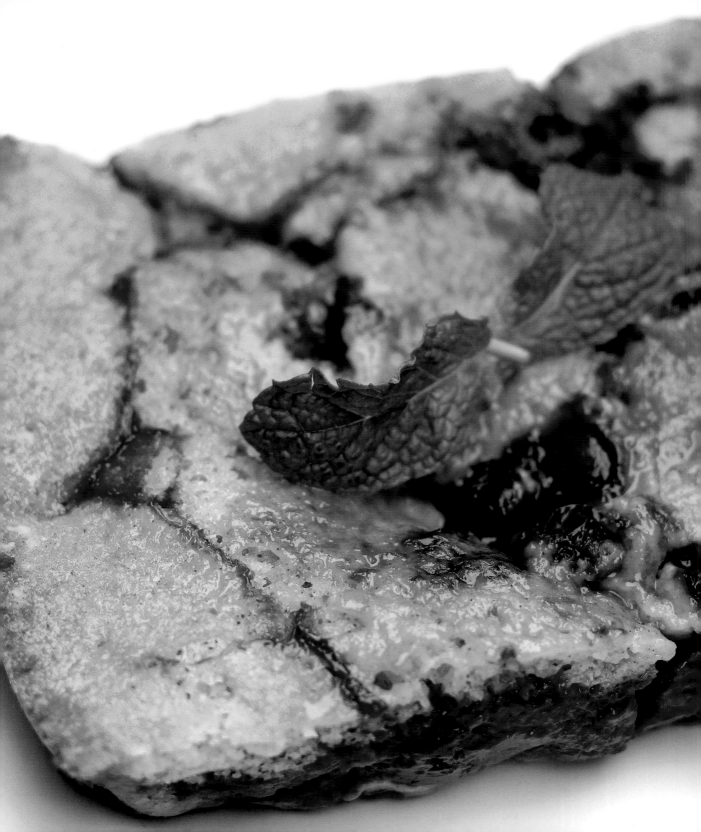

Dump Cake

Janice Muller, Derwood, MD

Makes 15 servings
Prep. Time: 20 minutes ⚹ Cooking Time: 50 minutes ⚹ Setting: Steam
Release: Manual ⚹ Cooling Time: 2–4 hours

20-ounce can crushed pineapple

21-ounce can light blueberry or cherry
pie filling

18½-ounce package yellow cake mix

Cinnamon

⅓ cup light, soft tub margarine

⅓ cup chopped walnuts

I cup water

Variation:

Use a package of spice cake mix and apple pie filling.

1. Grease bottom and sides of a 7" springform pan.

2. Spread layers of pineapple, blueberry pie filling, and dry cake mix. Be careful not to mix the layers.

3. Sprinkle with cinnamon.

4. Top with thin layers of margarine chunks and nuts.

5. Cover the pan with foil.

6. Place the trivet into your Instant Pot and pour in 1 cup of water. Place a foil sling on top of the trivet, then place the springform pan on top.

7. Secure the lid and make sure lid is set to sealing. Press Steam and set for 50 minutes.

8. When cook time is up, release the pressure manually, then carefully remove the springform pan by using hot pads to lift the pan up by the foil sling. Place on a cooling rack until cool.

Exchange List Values

Carbohydrate 2.5
Fat 1.0

Basic Nutritional Values

Calories 219 (Calories from Fat 57)
Total Fat 6 gm
(Saturated Fat 1.5 gm, Polyunsat Fat 2.4 gm, Monounsat Fat 2.2 gm)

Cholesterol 0 mg
Sodium 250 mg
Total Carb 41 gm
Dietary Fiber 1 gm
Sugars 28 gm
Protein 2 gm

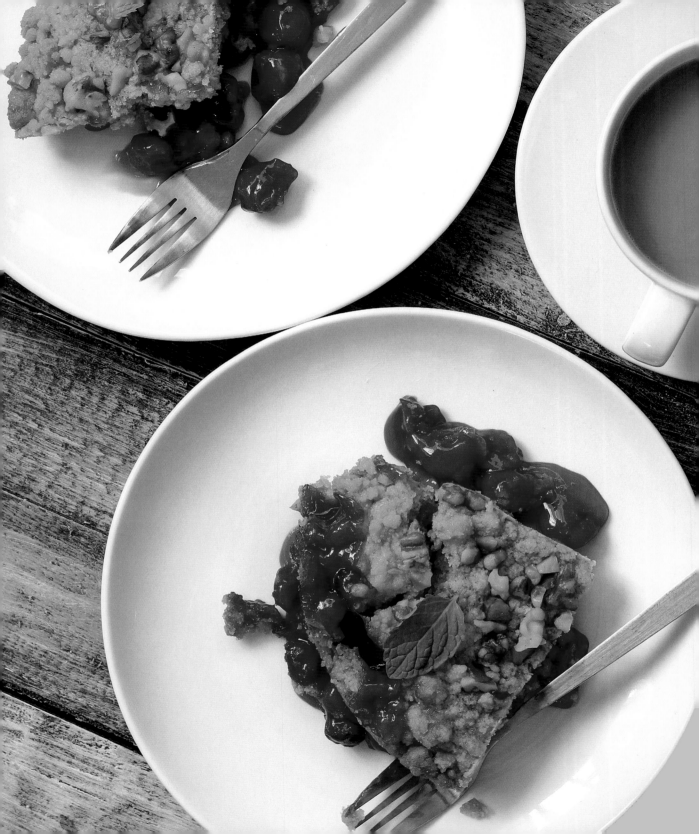

Cherry Delight

Anna Musser, Manheim, PA
Marianne J. Troyer, Millersburg, OH

Makes 12 servings
Prep. Time: 20 minutes ⚜ Cooking Time: 50 minutes ⚜ Setting: Steam
Release: Manual ⚜ Cooling Time: 1–2 hours

20-ounce can cherry pie filling, light
½ package yellow cake mix
¼ cup light, soft tub margarine, melted
⅓ cup walnuts, *optional*
1 cup water

1. Grease a 7" springform pan then pour the pie filing inside.

2. Combine dry cake mix and margarine (mixture will be crumbly) in a bowl. Sprinkle over filling. Sprinkle with walnuts.

3. Cover the pan with foil.

4. Place the trivet into your Instant Pot and pour in 1 cup of water. Place a foil sling on top of the trivet, then place the springform pan on top.

5. Secure the lid and make sure lid is set to sealing. Press Steam and set for 50 minutes.

6. When cook time is up, release the pressure manually, then carefully remove the springform pan by using hot pads to lift the pan up by the foil sling. Place on a cooling rack for 1–2 hours.

Serving suggestion:
Serve in bowls with dips of ice cream.

Exchange List Values

Carbohydrate 2.0

Basic Nutritional Values

Calories 137 (Calories from Fat 33)
Total Fat 4 gm
    (Saturated Fat 0.9 gm, Polyunsat Fat 0.9 gm, Monounsat Fat 1.6 gm)

Cholesterol 0 mg
Sodium 174 mg
Total Carb 26 gm
Dietary Fiber 1 gm
Sugars 19 gm
Protein 1 gm

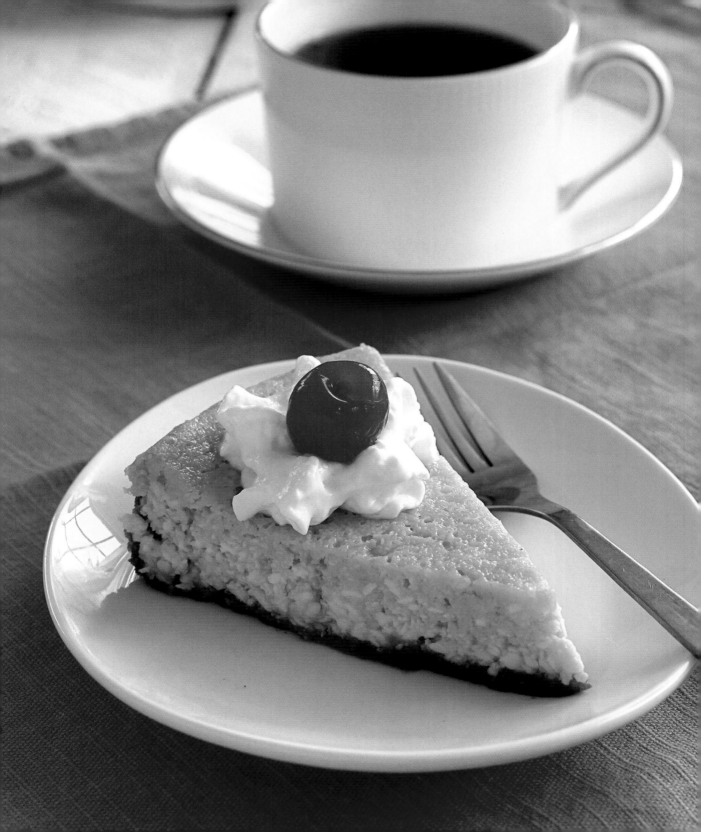

Creamy Orange Cheesecake

Jeanette Oberholtzer, Manheim, PA

Makes 10 servings

Prep. Time: 35 minutes ⚜ Cooking Time: 35 minutes ⚜ Setting: Manual ⚜ Pressure: High
Release: Natural then Manual ⚜ Cooling Time: 2 or more hours ⚜ Chilling Time: 4 or more hours

Crust:

¾ cup graham cracker crumbs

2 tablespoons sugar

3 tablespoons melted, light, soft tub margarine

Filling:

2 (8-ounce) packages fat-free cream cheese, at room temperature

⅔ cup sugar

2 eggs

1 egg yolk

¼ cup frozen orange juice concentrate

1 teaspoon orange zest

1 tablespoon flour

½ teaspoon vanilla

1½ cups water

1. Combine crust ingredients. Pat into 7" springform pan.

2. Cream together cream cheese and sugar. Add eggs and yolk. Beat for 3 minutes.

3. Beat in juice, zest, flour, and vanilla. Beat 2 minutes.

4. Pour batter into crust. Cover with foil.

5. Place the trivet into your Instant Pot and pour in 1½ cups water. Place a foil sling on top of the trivet, then place the springform pan on top.

6. Secure the lid and make sure lid is set to sealing. Press Manual and set for 35 minutes.

7. When cook time is up, press Cancel and allow the pressure to release naturally for 7 minutes, then release the remaining pressure manually.

8. Carefully remove the springform pan by using hot pads to lift the pan up by the foil sling. Uncover and place on a cooling rack until cool, then refrigerate for 8 hours.

Serving Suggestion:
Serve with thawed frozen whipped topping and fresh or mandarin orange slices.

Exchange List Values

Carbohydrate 1.5
Meat—lean 1.0

Basic Nutritional Values

Calories 159 (Calories from Fat 23)
Total Fat 3 gm (Saturated Fat 0.7 gm, Polyunsat Fat 0.6 gm, Monounsat Fat 1.1 gm)

Cholesterol 69 mg
Sodium 300 mg
Total Carb 25 gm
Dietary Fiber 0 gm
Sugars 19 gm
Protein 9 gm

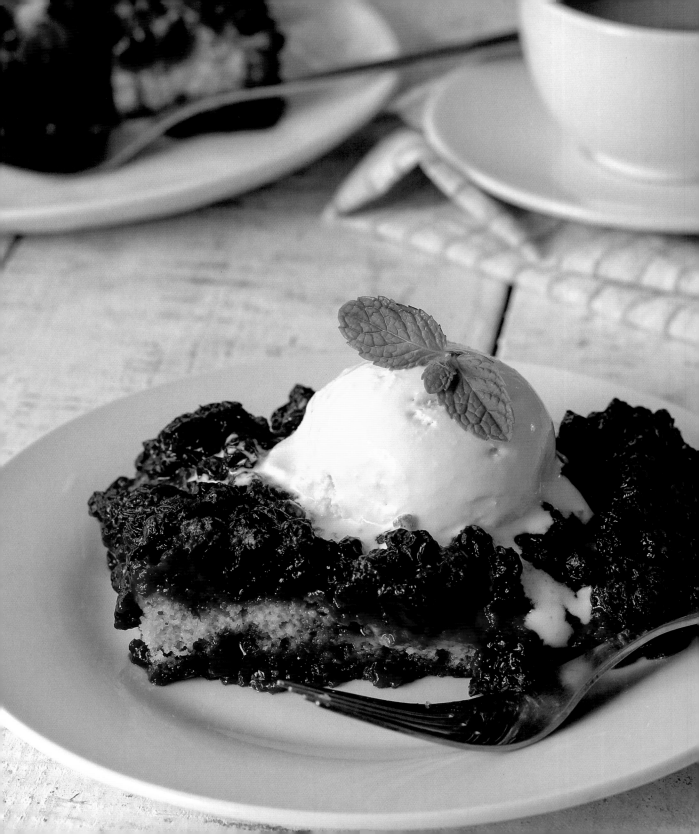

Black and Blue Cobbler

Renee Shirk, Mount Joy, PA

Makes 12 servings

Prep. Time: 30 minutes ⚜ Cooking Time: 15 minutes ⚜ Setting: Manual
Pressure: High ⚜ Release: Natural and Manual ⚜ Cooling Time: 30 minutes

1 cup flour

12 tablespoons sugar, *divided*

Sugar substitute to equal 6 tablespoons sugar, *divided*

1 teaspoon baking powder

¼ teaspoon salt

¼ teaspoon ground cinnamon

¼ teaspoon ground nutmeg

2 eggs, beaten

2 tablespoons milk

2 tablespoons vegetable oil

2 cups fresh, or frozen, blueberries

2 cups fresh, or frozen, blackberries

¾ cup water

1 teaspoon grated orange peel

1 cup water

Whipped topping or ice cream, *optional*

1. Combine flour, 6 Tbsp. sugar, sugar substitute equal to 3 Tbsp. sugar, baking powder, salt, cinnamon, and nutmeg.

2. Combine eggs, milk, and oil. Stir into dry ingredients until moistened.

3. Spread the batter evenly over bottom of greased 1½-quart baking dish.

4. In a saucepan, combine berries, water, orange peel, 6 Tbsp. sugar, and sugar substitute equal to 3 Tbsp. sugar. Bring to boil. Remove from heat and pour over batter. Cover with foil.

5. Place the trivet into your Instant Pot and pour in 1 cup of water. Place a foil sling on top of the trivet, then place the baking dish on top.

6. Secure the lid and make sure lid is set to sealing. Press Manual and set for 35 minutes.

7. When cook time is up, allow the pressure to release naturally for 10 minutes, then release the remaining pressure manually. Carefully remove the baking dish by using hot pads to lift the foil sling. Place on a cooling rack, uncovered for 30 minutes.

Serving suggestion:

Serve with whipped topping or ice cream, if desired.

Exchange List Values

Carbohydrate 2.0
Fat 0.5

Basic Nutritional Values

Calories 170 (Calories from Fat 31)
Total Fat 3 gm
    (Saturated Fat 0.5 gm, Polyunsat Fat 0.9 gm, Monounsat Fat 1.7 gm)

Cholesterol 36 mg
Sodium 92 mg
Total Carb 34 gm
Dietary Fiber 2 gm
Sugars 23 gm
Protein 3 gm

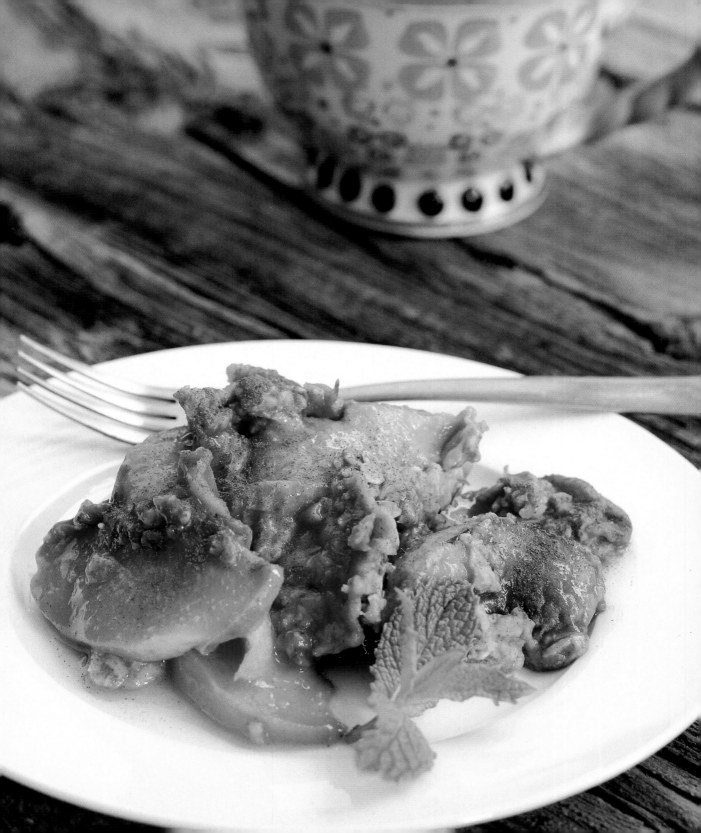

Quick Yummy Peaches

Willard E. Roth, Elkhart, IN

Makes 8 servings
Prep. Time: 20 minutes ⚜ Cooking Time: 20 minutes ⚜ Setting: Manual
Pressure: High ⚜ Release: Natural and Manual ⚜ Cooling Time: 20–30 minutes

⅓ cup buttermilk baking mix

⅔ cup dry quick oats

¼ cup brown sugar

Brown sugar substitute to equal 2 tablespoons sugar

1 teaspoon cinnamon

4 cups sliced peaches, canned or fresh

½ cup peach juice or water

1 cup water

1. Mix together baking mix, oats, brown sugar, brown sugar substitute, and cinnamon. Mix in the peaches and peach juice.

2. Pour mixture into a 1.6-quart baking dish. Cover with foil.

3. Place the trivet into your Instant Pot and pour in 1 cup of water. Place a foil sling on top of the trivet, then place the baking dish on top.

4. Secure the lid and make sure lid is set to sealing. Press Manual and set for 10 minutes.

5. When cook time is up, let the pressure release naturally for 10 minutes, then release any remaining pressure manually. Carefully remove the baking dish by using hot pads to lift the foil sling. Uncover and let cool for about 20–30 minutes.

Exchange List Values

Carbohydrate 2.0

Basic Nutritional Values

Calories 131 (Calories from Fat 11)
Total Fat 1 gm (Saturated Fat 0.1 gm, Polyunsat Fat 0.5 gm, Monounsat Fat 0.4 gm)

Cholesterol 0 mg
Sodium 76 mg
Total Carb 29 gm
Dietary Fiber 3 gm
Sugars 20 gm
Protein 2 gm

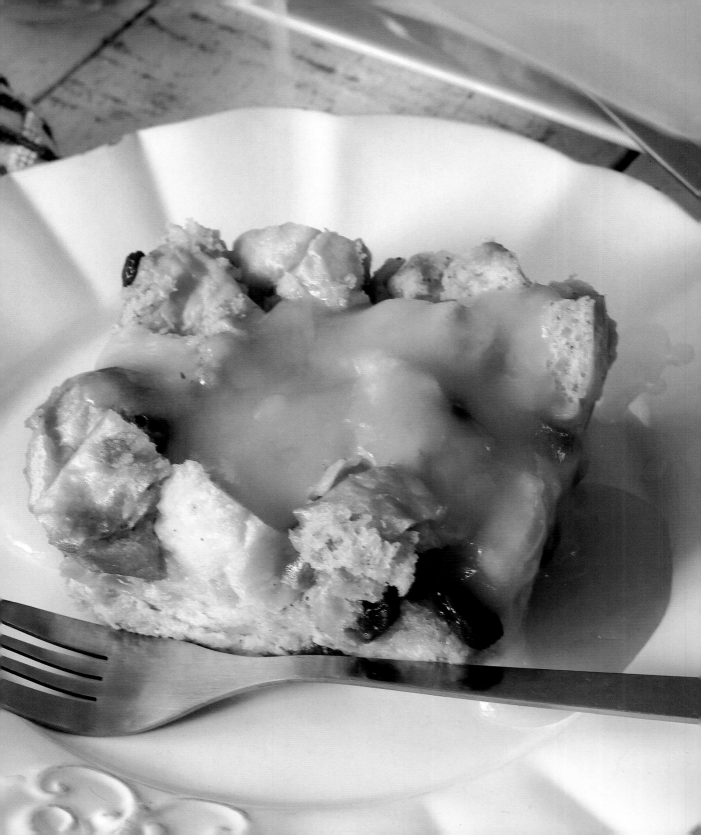

Bread Pudding

Winifred Ewy, Newton, KS
Helen King, Fairbank, IA
Elaine Patton, West Middletown, PA

Makes 9 servings
Prep. Time: 35 minutes ⚭ Cooking Time: 40 minutes ⚭ Setting: Manual
Pressure: High ⚭ Release: Natural and Manual

8 slices bread (raisin bread is especially good), cubed

3 eggs

2 egg whites

2 cups fat-free half-and-half

2 tablespoons sugar

Sugar substitute to equal 1 tablespoon sugar

½ cup raisins (use only ¼ cup if using raisin bread)

½ teaspoon cinnamon

1½ cups water

Sauce:

2 tablespoons light, soft tub margarine

2 tablespoons flour

1 cup water

6 tablespoons sugar

Sugar substitute to equal 3 tablespoons sugar

1 teaspoon vanilla

Serving Suggestion:

Serve sauce over warm bread pudding.

1. Place bread cubes in greased 1.6-quart baking dish.

2. Beat together eggs and half-and-half. Stir in sugar, sugar substitute, raisins, and cinnamon. Pour over bread and stir.

3. Cover with foil.

4. Place the trivet into your Instant Pot and pour in 1½ cups of water. Place a foil sling on top of the trivet, then place the baking dish on top.

5. Secure the lid and make sure lid is set to sealing. Press Manual and set time for 30 minutes.

6. When cook time is up, let the pressure release naturally for 15 minutes, then release any remaining pressure manually. Carefully remove the springform pan by using hot pads to lift the baking dish out by the foil sling. Let sit for a few minutes, uncovered, while you make the sauce.

7. Melt the margarine in saucepan. Stir in flour until smooth. Gradually add water, sugar, sugar substitute, and vanilla. Bring to a boil. Cook, stirring constantly for 2 minutes, or until thickened.

Exchange List Values

Carbohydrate 2.0
Fat 1.0

Basic Nutritional Values

Calories 200 (Calories from Fat 40)
Total Fat 4 gm (Saturated Fat 1.4 gm, Polyunsat Fat 0.6 gm, Monounsat Fat 1.7 gm)

Cholesterol 75 mg
Sodium 221 mg
Total Carb 34 gm
Dietary Fiber 1 gm
Sugars 21 gm
Protein 6 gm

Simple Bread Pudding

Melanie L. Thrower
McPherson, KS

Makes 8 servings
Prep. Time: 25 minutes   Cooking Time: 40 minutes   Setting: Manual
Pressure: High   Release: Natural and Manual

6–8 slices bread, cubed
2 cups fat-free milk
2 eggs
¼ cup sugar
I teaspoon ground cinnamon
I teaspoon vanilla
I ½ cups water

Sauce:
I tablespoon cornstarch
6-ounce can concentrated grape juice

1. Place bread cubes in greased 1.6-quart baking dish.

2. Beat together milk and eggs. Stir in sugar, cinnamon and vanilla. Pour over bread and stir.

3. Cover with foil.

4. Place the trivet into your Instant Pot and pour in 1½ cup of water. Place a foil sling on top of the trivet, then place the baking dish on top.

5. Secure the lid and make sure lid is set to sealing. Press Manual and set time for 30 minutes.

6. When cook time is up, let the pressure release naturally for 15 minutes, then release any remaining pressure manually. Carefully remove the springform pan by using hot pads to lift the baking dish out by the foil sling. Let sit for a few minutes, uncovered, while you make the sauce.

7. Combine cornstarch and concentrated juice in saucepan. Heat until boiling, stirring constantly, until sauce is thickened. Serve drizzled over bread pudding.

Exchange List Values

Carbohydrate 2.5

Basic Nutritional Values

Calories 179 (Calories from Fat 19)
Total Fat 2 gm (Saturated Fat 0.7 gm, Polyunsat Fat 0.6 gm, Monounsat Fat 0.6 gm)

Cholesterol 55 mg
Sodium 153 mg
Total Carb 35 gm
Dietary Fiber 1 gm
Sugars 24 gm
Protein 5 gm

Fruit Dessert Topping

Lavina Hochstedler, Grand Blanc, MI

Makes 40 (2 tablespoons) servings
Prep. Time: 15 minutes   Cooking Time: 3½–4 hours   Setting: Slow Cook and Sauté

3 tart apples, peeled and sliced

3 pears, peeled and sliced

1 tablespoon lemon juice

2 tablespoons brown sugar

Brown sugar substitute to equal 1 tablespoon sugar

2 tablespoons maple syrup

2 tablespoons light, soft tub margarine, melted

½ cup chopped pecans

¼ cup raisins

2 cinnamon sticks

1 tablespoon cornstarch

2 tablespoons cold water

1. Toss apples and pears in lemon juice in Instant Pot.

2. Combine brown sugar, brown sugar substitute, maple syrup, and margarine. Pour over fruit.

3. Stir in pecans, raisins, and cinnamon sticks.

4. Secure lid and press Slow Cook mode. Set on low 3–4 hours.

5. Combine cornstarch and water until smooth. Gradually stir into Instant Pot when cooking time is up.

6. Press Sauté and continue to cook until sauce is thickened, stirring frequently.

7. Discard cinnamon sticks.

Serving Suggestion:

1. Serve over pound cake or ice cream.

2. We also like this served along with pancakes or an egg casserole. We always use Fruit Dessert Topping for our breakfasts at church camp.

Exchange List Values

Carbohydrate 0.5

Basic Nutritional Values

Calories 33 (Calories from Fat 13)

Total Fat 1 gm (Saturated Fat 0.1 gm, Polyunsat Fat 0.4 gm, Monounsat Fat 0.8 gm)

Cholesterol 0 mg

Sodium 5 mg

Total Carb 6 gm

Dietary Fiber 1 gm

Sugars 5 gm

Protein 0 gm

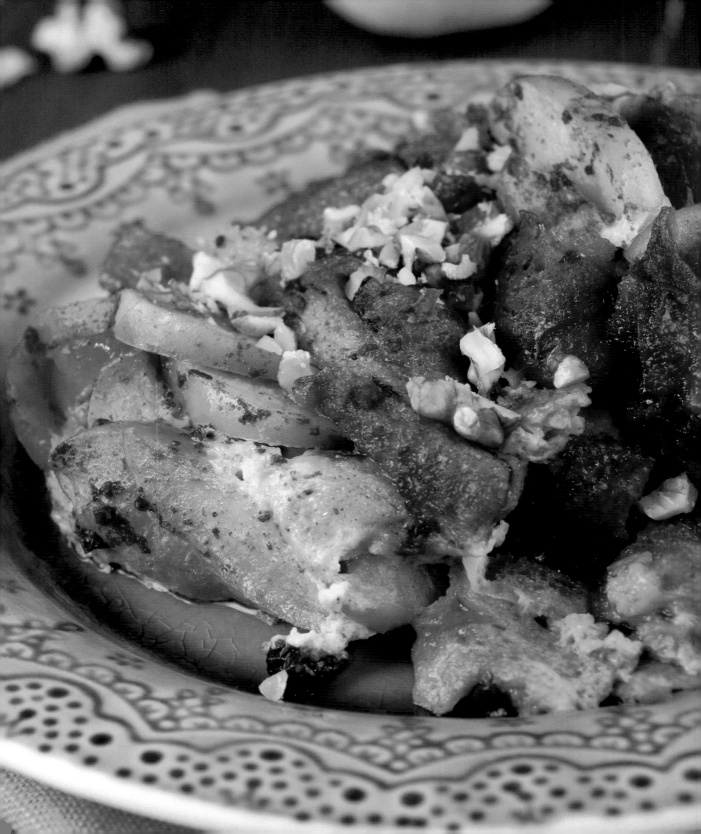

Apple-Nut Bread Pudding

Ruth Ann Hoover, New Holland, PA

Makes 10 servings
Prep. Time: 20 minutes ⚜ Cooking Time: 40 minutes ⚜ Setting: Manual
Pressure: High ⚜ Release: Natural and Manual

8 slices raisin bread, cubed

2 medium-sized tart apples, peeled and sliced

1 cup chopped pecans, toasted

½ cup sugar

Sugar substitute to equal ¼ cup sugar

1 teaspoon ground cinnamon

½ teaspoon ground nutmeg

1 egg, lightly beaten

3 egg whites, lightly beaten

2 cups fat-free half-and-half

¼ cup apple juice

2 tablespoons light, soft tub margarine, melted

1. Place bread cubes, apples, and pecans in greased 1.6-quart baking dish and mix gently.

2. Combine sugar, sugar substitute, cinnamon, and nutmeg. Add remaining ingredients. Mix well. Pour over bread mixture.

3. Cover with foil.

4. Place the trivet into your Instant Pot and pour in 1½ cup of water. Place a foil sling on top of the trivet, then place the baking dish on top.

5. Secure the lid and make sure lid is set to sealing. Press Manual and set time for 30 minutes.

6. When cook time is up, let the pressure release naturally for 15 minutes, then release any remaining pressure manually. Carefully remove the springform pan by using hot pads to lift the baking dish out by the foil sling.

Exchange List Values

Carbohydrate 2.0
Fat 2.0

Basic Nutritional Values

Calories 231 (Calories from Fat 87)
Total Fat 10 gm (Saturated Fat 1.4 gm, Polyunsat Fat 2.3 gm, Monounsat Fat 5.1 gm)

Cholesterol 25 mg
Sodium 191 mg
Total Carb 32 gm
Dietary Fiber 2 gm
Sugars 20 gm
Protein 6 gm

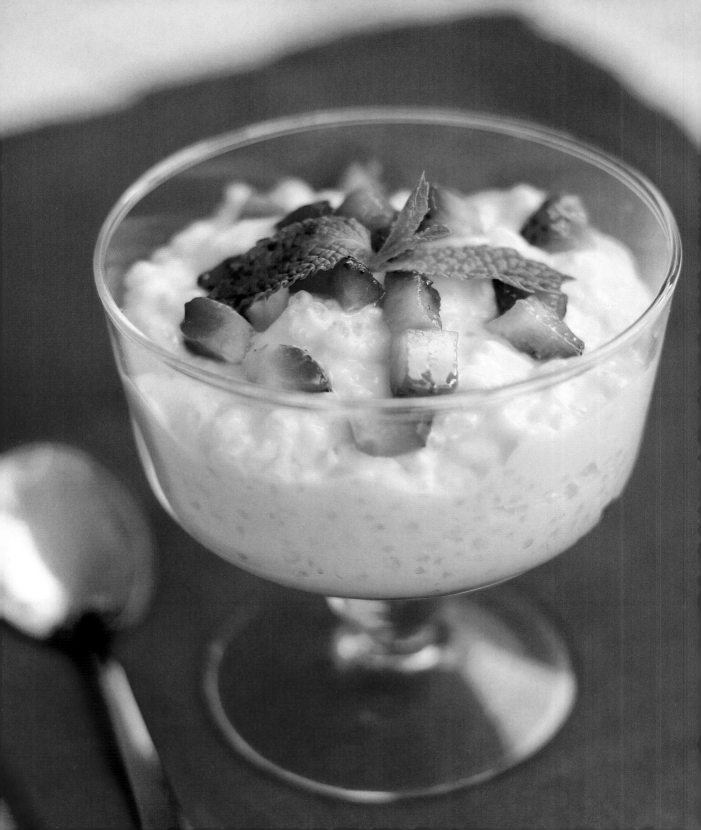

Instant Pot Tapioca

Nancy W. Huber, Green Park, PA

Makes 6 servings
Prep. Time: 10 minutes ⚜ Cooking Time: 7 minutes ⚜ Setting: Manual
Pressure: High ⚜ Release: Manual

2 cups water
I cup small pearl tapioca
½ cup sugar
4 eggs
½ cup evaporated skim milk
Sugar substitute to equal ¼ cup sugar
I teaspoon vanilla
Fruit of choice, *optional*

1. Combine water and tapioca in Instant Pot.

2. Secure lid and make sure vent is set to sealing. Press Manual and set for 5 minutes.

3. Perform a quick release. Press Cancel, remove lid, and press Sauté.

4. Whisk together eggs and evaporated milk. SLOWLY add to the Instant Pot, stirring constantly so the eggs don't scramble.

5. Stir in the sugar substitute until it's dissolved, press Cancel, then stir in the vanilla.

6. Allow to cool thoroughly, then refrigerate at least 4 hours.

Serving suggestion:

Serve with fruit.

Exchange List Values

Carbohydrate 3.5
Fat 0.5

Basic Nutritional Values

Calories 262 (Calories from Fat 27)
Total Fat 3 gm
   (Saturated Fat 1.1 gm, Polyunsat Fat 0.6 gm, Monounsat Fat 1.2 gm)

Cholesterol 124 mg
Sodium 75 mg
Total Carb 50 gm
Dietary Fiber 0 gm
Sugars 28 gm
Protein 6 gm

Wine-Poached Pears

Hope Comerford, Clinton Township, MI

Makes 6 servings
Prep. Time: 20 minutes & Cooking Time: 10 minutes & Setting: Manual and Sauté
Pressure: High & Release: Natural and Manual

1 bottle red blend wine

1 cup Truvia brown sugar blend

1 teaspoon grated lemon peel

6 fresh pears, peeled, but stem attached

2 cinnamon sticks

1. In the Instant Pot, mix together the wine, brown sugar blend and lemon peel.

2. Place the pears and cinnamon sticks into the liquid inside the Instant Pot.

3. Secure the lid and make sure the vent is set to sealing. Press Manual and set time for 5 minutes.

4. Let the pressure release naturally for 10 minutes, then perform a quick release.

5. Remove the lid and carefully remove the pears with tongs and set aside.

6. Press Sauté and continue to cook until the sauce has reduced to a third of the original amount.

Serving suggestion:

Serve pears at room temperature or chilled with the sauce drizzled over the top.

Exchange List Values

Fruit 4

Basic Nutritional Values

Calories 368 (Calories from Fat 2)
Total Fat .2 gm (Saturated Fat 0 gm, Polyunsat Fat 0.2 gm, Monounsat Fat 0.1 gm)

Cholesterol 0 mg
Sodium 2 mg
Total Carb 62 gm
Dietary Fiber 5 gm
Sugars 48 gm
Protein 1 gm

Scalloped Pineapples

Shirley Hinh, Wayland, IA

Makes 8 servings
Prep. Time: 15 minutes ⚓ *Cooking Time: 3 hours* ⚓ *Setting: Slow Cook*

½ cup sugar

Sugar substitute to equal ¼ cup sugar

3 eggs

¼ cup light, soft margarine, melted

¾ cup milk

20-ounce can crushed pineapple, drained

8 slices bread (crusts removed), cubed

1. Mix together all ingredients in the Instant Pot.

2. Secure the lid and set to Slow Cook mode on high for 2 hours. Reduce heat to low and cook 1 more hour.

Exchange List Values

Carbohydrate 2.0
Fat 0.5

Basic Nutritional Values

Calories 181 (Calories from Fat 44)
Total Fat 5 gm (Saturated Fat 1.1 gm, Polyunsat Fat 1.1 gm, Monounsat Fat 2.1 gm)

Cholesterol 81 mg
Sodium 176 mg
Total Carb 30 gm
Dietary Fiber 1 gm
Sugars 21 gm
Protein 5 gm

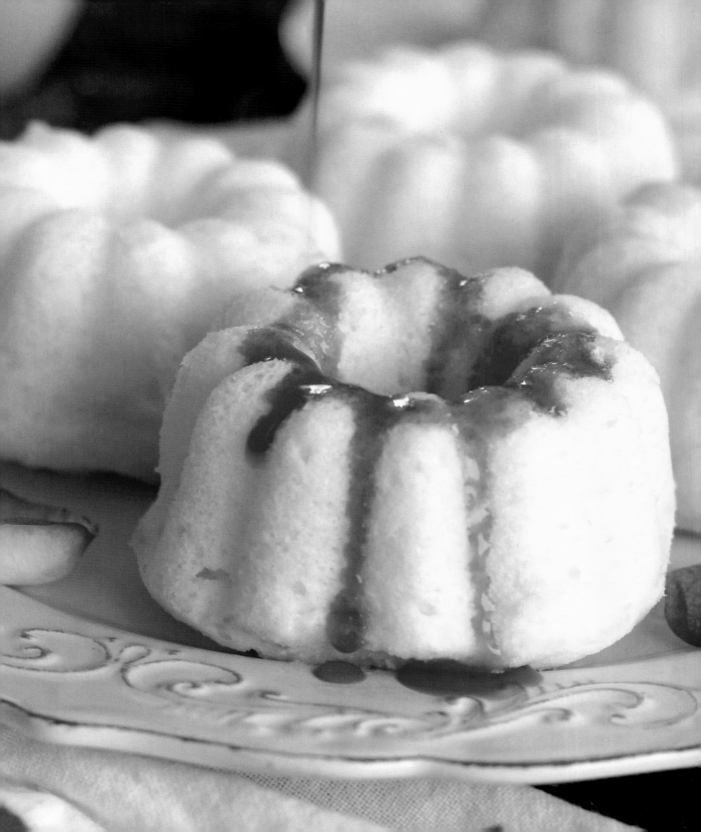

Rhubarb Sauce

Esther Porter, Minneapolis, MN

Makes 6 servings
Prep. Time: 20 minutes   ⚭   Cooking Time: 4–5 hours
Chilling Time: 4 hours minimum   ⚭   Setting: Slow Cook

1 ½ **pounds rhubarb**
⅛ **teaspoon salt**
½ **cup water**
½ **cup sugar**

1. Cut rhubarb into ½-inch slices.

2. Combine all ingredients in Instant Pot. Press Slow Cook mode and cook on low 4–5 hours.

3. Serve chilled.

Variation:

Add 1 pint sliced strawberries about 30 minutes before removing from heat.

Exchange List Values

Carbohydrate 1.0

Basic Nutritional Values

Calories 80 (Calories from Fat 1)
Total Fat 0 gm
(Saturated Fat 0.0 gm, Polyunsat Fat 0.0 gm, Monounsat Fat 0.0 gm)

Cholesterol 0 mg
Sodium 54 mg
Total Carb 20 gm
Dietary Fiber 2 gm
Sugars 17 gm
Protein 1 gm

Metric Equivalent Measurements

If you're accustomed to using metric measurements, I don't want you to be inconvenienced by the imperial measurements I use in this book.

Use this handy chart, too, to figure out the size of the slow cooker you'll need for each recipe.

Weight (Dry Ingredients)

1 oz		30 g
4 oz	¼ lb	120 g
8 oz	½ lb	240 g
12 oz	¾ lb	360 g
16 oz	1 lb	480 g
32 oz	2 lb	960 g

Slow Cooker Sizes

1-quart	0.96 l
2-quart	1.92 l
3-quart	2.88 l
4-quart	3.84 l
5-quart	4.80 l
6-quart	5.76 l
7-quart	6.72 l
8-quart	7.68 l

Volume (Liquid Ingredients)

½ tsp.		2 ml
1 tsp.		5 ml
1 Tbsp.	½ fl oz	15 ml
2 Tbsp.	1 fl oz	30 ml
¼ cup	2 fl oz	60 ml
⅓ cup	3 fl oz	80 ml
½ cup	4 fl oz	120 ml
⅔ cup	5 fl oz	160 ml
¾ cup	6 fl oz	180 ml
1 cup	8 fl oz	240 ml
1 pt	16 fl oz	480 ml
1 qt	32 fl oz	960 ml

Length

¼ in	6 mm
½ in	13 mm
¾ in	19 mm
1 in	25 mm
6 in	15 cm
12 in	30 cm

Recipe and Ingredient Index

A

almonds
    Best Steel Cut-Oats, 35
Ann's Chicken Cacciatore, 129
apple
    Fruit Dessert Topping, 243
apple juice
    Apple Walnut Squash, 194
Apple Oatmeal, 31
Apple Walnut Squash, 194
artichoke hearts
    Spinach and Artichoke Dip, 49
Artichokes, 61
Asian Pepper Steak, 167

B

bacon
    Baked Navy Beans, 221
    Baked Pinto Beans, 219
    Potato-Bacon Gratin, 25
    Potato Bacon Soup, 79
bacon bits
    Easy Quiche, 24
Baked Acorn Squash, 193
Baked Eggs, 23
Baked Navy Beans, 221
Baked Pinto Beans, 219
barbecue sauce
    BBQ Pork Sandwiches, 187
    Pulled Pork, 185
    Tender Tasty Ribs, 183
barley
    Beef Roast with Mushroom Barley, 161
Bavarian Beef, 165
BBQ Pork Sandwiches, 187
beans
    black
        Black Bean Soup, 87
        Ground Turkey Stew, 93
        Southwestern Bean Soup with Corn
            Dumplings, 85
        Three-Bean Chili, 109
    cannellini
        Tuscan Beef Stew, 101
    chili
        Favorite Chili, 111
        Pizza in a Pot, 145
    French Market Soup, 75
    garbanzo
        Chicken Casablanca, 127
        Hummus, 43
        Vegetable Curry, 199
    garbanzo beans
        Hummus, 43
    great northern
        Old Fashioned Ham 'n' Beans, 223
        White Chicken Chili, 105
    green
        Nancy's Vegetable Beef Soup, 71
        "Smothered" Steak, 171
        Vegetable Curry, 199
    kidney
        Italian Vegetable Soup, 82
        Southwestern Bean Soup with Corn
            Dumplings, 85
        Three-Bean Chili, 109
        Turkey Chili, 107
    navy
        Baked Navy Beans, 221
    pinto
        Baked Pinto Beans, 219
        Turkey Chili, 107
beef
    Asian Pepper Steak, 167
    Bavarian Beef, 165
    Beef Burgundy, 159
    Beef Dumpling Soup, 74
    Easy Pot Roast and Vegetables, 157
    Favorite Chili, 111
    Garlic Beef Stroganoff, 175
    Instantly Good Beef Stew, 99
    Machaca Beef, 163
    Nancy's Vegetable Beef Soup, 71
    Pot Roast, 153

Pot Roast with Gravy and Vegetables, 155
Pot Roast with Tomato Sauce, 154
Quick Steak Tacos, 177
Smokey Barbecue Meatballs, 57
"Smothered" Steak, 171
Steak Stroganoff, 173
Three-Bean Chili, 109
Three-Pepper Steak, 169
Tuscan Beef Stew, 101
Zesty Swiss Steak, 166
Beef Broccoli, 179
Beef Burgundy, 159
Beef Dumpling Soup, 74
Beef Roast with Mushroom Barley, 161
Beef Stew, 96–97, 99, 101
bell pepper
    Asian Pepper Steak, 167
    Cheesy Stuffed Cabbage, 149
    Chicken Cheddar Broccoli Soup, 65
    Italian Wild Mushrooms, 205
    Janie's Vegetable Medley, 195
    Pot Roast with Gravy and Vegetables, 155
    "Smothered" Steak, 171
    Szechuan-Style Chicken and Broccoli, 133
    Taylor's Favorite Uniquely Stuffed Peppers,
        147
    Turkey Sloppy Joes, 151
    Vegetable Curry, 199
    Vegetarian Chili, 113
Best Brown Rice, 197
Best Steel Cut-Oats, 35
biscuits
    Beef Dumpling Soup, 74
Black and Blue Cobbler, 237
Black Bean Soup, 87
blackberries
    Black and Blue Cobbler, 237
Blackberry Baked Brie, 45
blueberries
    Black and Blue Cobbler, 237
blueberry pie filling
    Dump Cake, 231
bread
    Cinnamon French Toast, 15
    French Onion Soup, 81
    Simple Bread Pudding, 242
    Stewed Tomatoes, 207
    Turkey Sloppy Joes, 151
Bread Pudding, 241, 242

broccoli
    Beef Broccoli, 179
    Chicken Cheddar Broccoli Soup, 65
    Szechuan-Style Chicken and Broccoli, 133
Brown Lentil Soup, 89
Brown Rice, 217
Buffalo Chicken Dip, 53
Butternut Squash Soup, 91
Buttery Lemon Chicken, 121

C
cabbage
    Cheesy Stuffed Cabbage, 149
    Chicken Vegetable Soup, 70
    Unstuffed Cabbage Soup, 73
cake mix
    Cherry Delight, 233
Candied Pecans, 41
Caramelized Onions, 203
carrot
    Beef Dumpling Soup, 74
    Chicken Cheddar Broccoli Soup, 65
    Italian Vegetable Soup, 82
    Simple Salted Carrots, 201
    Vegetable Curry, 199
    Vegetable Medley, 196
Carrot Cake, 229
cheese
    Brie
        Blackberry Baked Brie, 45
    cheddar
        Buffalo Chicken Dip, 53
        Cheesy Stuffed Cabbage, 149
        Chicken Cheddar Broccoli Soup, 65
        Creamy Jalapeño Chicken Dip, 51
        Easy Quiche, 24
        Potato-Bacon Gratin, 25
        Potato Bacon Soup, 79
        Shredded Potato Omelet, 29
        Southwestern Egg Casserole, 27
    cottage
        Southwestern Egg Casserole, 27
    Mexi-blend
        White Chicken Chili, 105
    Mexican
        Quick Steak Tacos, 177
    Monterey Jack
        Creamy Spinach Dip, 47

mozzarella
    Cheesy Stuffed Cabbage, 149
    Spinach and Artichoke Dip, 49
  Parmesan
    Cheesy Stuffed Cabbage, 149
    Creamy Spinach Dip, 47
    Pizza in a Pot, 145
    Spinach and Artichoke Dip, 49
  Swiss
    Chicken Reuben Bake, 139
    Potato-Bacon Gratin, 25
Cheesy Stuffed Cabbage, 149
cherries, dried
  Best Steel Cut-Oats, 35
Cherry Delight, 233
cherry pie filling
  Dump Cake, 231
chicken
  Ann's Chicken Cacciatore, 129
  Buffalo Chicken Dip, 53
  Buttery Lemon Chicken, 121
  Creamy Chicken Wild Rice Soup, 67
  Creamy Jalapeño Chicken Dip, 51
  Creamy Nutmeg Chicken, 140
  Garlic Galore Rotisserie Chicken, 119
  Greek Chicken, 125
  Lemony Chicken Thighs, 135
  Mild Chicken Curry with Coconut Milk, 143
  Orange Chicken Thighs with Bell Peppers, 137
  Szechuan-Style Chicken and Broccoli, 133
  White Chicken Chili, 105
Chicken Casablanca, 127
Chicken Cheddar Broccoli Soup, 65
Chicken in Mushroom Gravy, 141
Chicken in Wine, 123
Chicken Reuben Bake, 139
Chicken Rice Soup, 69
Chicken Vegetable Soup, 70
chicken wings
  Levi's Sesame Chicken Wings, 55
Chicken with Spiced Sesame Sauce, 131
chickpeas
  Hummus, 43
Cinnamon French Toast, 15
coconut milk
  Mild Chicken Curry with Coconut Milk, 143
corn
  Chicken Vegetable Soup, 70
  Easy Southern Brunswick Stew, 103
  Nancy's Vegetable Beef Soup, 71
Corn on the Cob, 202
cranberries
  Oatmeal Morning, 33
cream cheese
  Buffalo Chicken Dip, 53
  Creamy Chicken Wild Rice Soup, 67
  Creamy Jalapeño Chicken Dip, 51
  Creamy Orange Cheesecake, 235
  Creamy Spinach Dip, 47
  Garlic Beef Stroganoff, 175
  Spinach and Artichoke Dip, 49
cream of mushroom soup
  Chicken in Mushroom Gravy, 141
  Chicken in Wine, 123
  Creamy Nutmeg Chicken, 140
  Garlic Beef Stroganoff, 175
  Steak Stroganoff, 173
  Turkey Meatballs and Gravy, 144
Creamy Chicken Wild Rice Soup, 67
Creamy Jalapeño Chicken Dip, 51
Creamy Nutmeg Chicken, 140
Creamy Orange Cheesecake, 235
Creamy Spinach Dip, 47
Cynthia's Yogurt, 17

D
dates
  Carrot Cake, 229
Dump Cake, 231
dumplings
  Southwestern Bean Soup with Corn Dumplings, 85

E
Easy Pot Roast and Vegetables, 157
Easy Quiche, 24
Easy Southern Brunswick Stew, 103
eggs
  Easy Quiche, 24
  Instant Pot Hard-Boiled Eggs, 21, 23
  Poached Eggs, 19

F
Favorite Chili, 111
French Market Soup, 75
French onion soup
  Chicken in Wine, 123

French Onion Soup, 81
Fruit Dessert Topping, 243

G
Garlic Beef Stroganoff, 175
Garlic Galore Rotisserie Chicken, 119
ginger
    Chicken with Spiced Sesame Sauce, 131
graham crackers
    Creamy Orange Cheesecake, 235
gravy mix
    Pot Roast with Gravy and Vegetables, 155
Greek Chicken, 125
Green Chile Corn Chowder, 95
green chiles
    Green Chile Corn Chowder, 95
    Machaca Beef, 163
    Pork Chili, 83
    Southwestern Bean Soup with Corn
        Dumplings, 85
    Southwestern Egg Casserole, 27
    White Chicken Chili, 105
green pepper
    Shredded Potato Omelet, 29
Ground Turkey Stew, 93

H
ham
    Green Chile Corn Chowder, 95
    Ham and Potato Chowder, 115
    Italian Vegetable Soup, 82
    Old Fashioned Ham 'n' Beans, 223
    Split Pea Soup, 77
Ham and Potato Chowder, 115
honey
    Apple Oatmeal, 31
Honey Lemon Garlic Salmon, 189
hot sauce
    Buffalo Chicken Dip, 53
    Chicken Cheddar Broccoli Soup, 65
    Janie's Vegetable Medley, 195
    Nancy's Vegetable Beef Soup, 71
Hummus, 43

I
Instantly Good Beef Stew, 99
Instant Pot Hard-Boiled Eggs, 21
Insta Popcorn, 39
Italian Vegetable Soup, 82
Italian Wild Mushrooms, 205

J
jalapeño
    Creamy Jalapeño Chicken Dip, 51
    Three-Pepper Steak, 169
    Vegetarian Chili, 113
Janie's Vegetable Medley, 195

K
ketchup
    Baked Pinto Beans, 219
    Easy Southern Brunswick Stew, 103
    Levi's Sesame Chicken Wings, 55
    Smokey Barbecue Meatballs, 57
    Turkey Sloppy Joes, 151

L
Lemon Pudding Cake, 227
Lemony Chicken Thighs, 135
lentils
    Brown Lentil Soup, 89
Levi's Sesame Chicken Wings, 55
lima beans
    Chicken Vegetable Soup, 70

M
Machaca Beef, 163
maple syrup
    Cinnamon French Toast, 15
Mashed Potatoes, 215
Mild Chicken Curry with Coconut
    Milk, 143
mushrooms
    Ann's Chicken Cacciatore, 129
    Asian Pepper Steak, 167
    Beef Burgundy, 159
    Beef Roast with Mushroom Barley, 161
    Beef Stew, 96–97
    Cheesy Stuffed Cabbage, 149
    Chicken in Mushroom Gravy, 141
    Creamy Chicken Wild Rice Soup, 67
    Easy Quiche, 24
    Garlic Beef Stroganoff, 175
    Italian Wild Mushrooms, 205
    "Smothered" Steak, 171
mustard
    Baked Pinto Beans, 219
    Bavarian Beef, 165
    Turkey Sloppy Joes, 151

N

Nancy's Vegetable Beef Soup, 71

O

Oatmeal Morning, 33
oats
    Apple Oatmeal, 31
    Best Steel Cut-Oats, 35
    Quick Yummy Peaches, 239
    Smokey Barbecue Meatballs, 57
    Taylor's Favorite Uniquely Stuffed Peppers,
       147
Old Fashioned Ham 'n' Beans, 223
onions
    Caramelized Onions, 203
    French Onion Soup, 81
onion soup mix
    Easy Pot Roast and Vegetables, 157
    Steak Stroganoff, 173
Orange Chicken Thighs with Bell Peppers, 137
orange juice
    Baked Acorn Squash, 193
orange spread
    Orange Chicken Thighs with Bell
       Peppers, 137

P

parsnip
    Vegetable Medley, 196
peaches
    Quick Yummy Peaches, 239
pears
    Fruit Dessert Topping, 243
peas
    Beef Stew, 96–97
    Chicken Vegetable Soup, 70
    Easy Southern Brunswick Stew, 103
    Janie's Vegetable Medley, 195
    Nancy's Vegetable Beef Soup, 71
    split
       Split Pea Soup, 77
pecans
    Baked Acorn Squash, 193
    Candied Pecans, 41
    Fruit Dessert Topping, 243
Perfect Sweet Potatoes, 211
pickles
    Bavarian Beef, 165

pie filling
    Cherry Delight, 233
    Dump Cake, 231
pimento
    Green Chile Corn Chowder, 95
pineapple
    Dump Cake, 231
Pizza in a Pot, 145
Poached Eggs, 19
popcorn
    Insta Popcorn, 39
Porcupine Meatballs, 59
pork
    BBQ Pork Sandwiches, 187
    Pulled Pork, 185
pork butt
    Easy Southern Brunswick Stew, 103
Pork Butt Roast, 181
Pork Chili, 83
pork ribs
    Pork Chili, 83
Potato-Bacon Gratin, 25
Potato Bacon Soup, 79
potatoes
    Beef Stew, 96–97
    Chicken Casablanca, 127
    Chicken Vegetable Soup, 70
    Easy Pot Roast and Vegetables, 157
    Greek Chicken, 125
    Green Chile Corn Chowder, 95
    Ham and Potato Chowder, 115
    Instantly Good Beef Stew, 99
    Italian Vegetable Soup, 82
    Janie's Vegetable Medley, 195
    Mashed Potatoes, 215
    Potato-Bacon Gratin, 25
    Pot Roast, 153
    Pot Roast with Gravy and Vegetables, 155
    Pot Roast with Tomato Sauce, 154
    Shredded Potato Omelet, 29
    Vegetable Curry, 199
Potatoes with Parsley, 213
Pot Roast, 153
Pot Roast with Gravy and Vegetables, 155
Pot Roast with Tomato Sauce, 154
Pulled Pork, 185

Q

Quick Steak Tacos, 177

Quick Yummy Peaches, 239

R

raisins
    Best Steel Cut-Oats, 35
    Bread Pudding, 241
    Chicken Casablanca, 127
    Fruit Dessert Topping, 243
ranch dressing
    Buffalo Chicken Dip, 53
ribs
    Pork Chili, 83
    Tender Tasty Ribs, 183
rice
    brown
        Best Brown Rice, 197
        Brown Rice, 217
        Porcupine Meatballs, 59
        Unstuffed Cabbage Soup, 73
    Chicken Rice Soup, 69
    Janie's Vegetable Medley, 195
    wild
        Chicken Rice Soup, 69
        Creamy Chicken Wild Rice Soup, 67

S

salmon
    Honey Lemon Garlic Salmon, 189
salsa
    Machaca Beef, 163
    Quick Steak Tacos, 177
    Three-Bean Chili, 109
sauerkraut
    Chicken Reuben Bake, 139
sausage
    Pizza in a Pot, 145
    Taylor's Favorite Uniquely Stuffed Peppers,
        147
Shredded Potato Omelet, 29
Simple Bread Pudding, 242
Simple Salted Carrots, 201
Smokey Barbecue Meatballs, 57
"Smothered" Steak, 171
sour cream
    Black Bean Soup, 87
    Creamy Jalapeño Chicken Dip, 51
    Creamy Nutmeg Chicken, 140
    Creamy Spinach Dip, 47
    Potato Bacon Soup, 79

Quick Steak Tacos, 177
    Spinach and Artichoke Dip, 49
    Steak Stroganoff, 173
    White Chicken Chili, 105
Southwestern Bean Soup with Corn
    Dumplings, 85
Southwestern Egg Casserole, 27
soy sauce
    Asian Pepper Steak, 167
    Beef Broccoli, 179
    Levi's Sesame Chicken Wings, 55
    "Smothered" Steak, 171
    Szechuan-Style Chicken and Broccoli, 133
spinach
    Creamy Spinach Dip, 47
    Potato-Bacon Gratin, 25
Spinach and Artichoke Dip, 49
Split Pea Soup, 77
squash
    Apple Walnut Squash, 194
    Baked Acorn Squash, 193
    Butternut Squash Soup, 91
Steak Stroganoff, 173
Stewed Tomatoes, 207
sweet potato
    Chicken Vegetable Soup, 70
    Perfect Sweet Potatoes, 211
Sweet Potato Puree, 209
Szechuan-Style Chicken and Broccoli, 133

T

tahini
    Chicken with Spiced Sesame Sauce, 131
    Hummus, 43
tapioca
    Pizza in a Pot, 145
    Szechuan-Style Chicken and Broccoli, 133
    Vegetable Curry, 199
Taylor's Favorite Uniquely Stuffed Peppers, 147
Tender Tasty Ribs, 183
textured vegetable protein
    Vegetarian Chili, 113
Thousand Island dressing
    Chicken Reuben Bake, 139
Three-Bean Chili, 109
Three-Pepper Steak, 169
tomatoes
    Chicken Casablanca, 127
    Chicken Vegetable Soup, 70

Favorite Chili, 111
French Market Soup, 75
Ground Turkey Stew, 93
Italian Vegetable Soup, 82
Italian Wild Mushrooms, 205
Janie's Vegetable Medley, 195
Mild Chicken Curry with Coconut Milk, 143
Nancy's Vegetable Beef Soup, 71
Pizza in a Pot, 145
Pork Chili, 83
"Smothered" Steak, 171
Southwestern Bean Soup with Corn
    Dumplings, 85
Stewed Tomatoes, 207
Three-Bean Chili, 109
Three-Pepper Steak, 169
Turkey Chili, 107
Tuscan Beef Stew, 101
Vegetable Curry, 199
Vegetarian Chili, 113
Zesty Swiss Steak, 166
tomato sauce
    Cheesy Stuffed Cabbage, 149
    Ground Turkey Stew, 93
    Instantly Good Beef Stew, 99
tomato soup
    Easy Southern Brunswick Stew, 103
    Porcupine Meatballs, 59
    Tuscan Beef Stew, 101
tortillas
    Quick Steak Tacos, 177
turkey
    Cheesy Stuffed Cabbage, 149
    Ground Turkey Stew, 93
    Porcupine Meatballs, 59
    Taylor's Favorite Uniquely Stuffed Peppers,
        147
    Unstuffed Cabbage Soup, 73
Turkey Chili, 107
Turkey Meatballs and Gravy, 144

turkey sausage
    Pizza in a Pot, 145
Turkey Sloppy Joes, 151
Tuscan Beef Stew, 101

U
Unstuffed Cabbage Soup, 73

V
Vegetable Curry, 199
Vegetable Medley, 196
Vegetarian Chili, 113
vinegar
    red wine
        Chicken with Spiced Sesame Sauce, 131

W
walnuts
    Apple Oatmeal, 31
    Apple Walnut Squash, 194
    Cherry Delight, 233
    Dump Cake, 231
    Oatmeal Morning, 33
White Chicken Chili, 105

Y
yogurt
    Black Bean Soup, 87
    Cynthia's Yogurt, 17
    Southwestern Bean Soup with Corn
        Dumplings, 85

Z
Zesty Swiss Steak, 166
zucchini
    Chicken Casablanca, 127
    Janie's Vegetable Medley, 195
    Taylor's Favorite Uniquely Stuffed
        Peppers, 147

About the Author

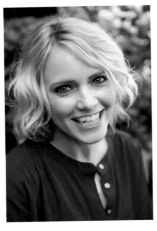

Hope Comerford is a mom, wife, elementary music teacher, blogger, recipe developer, public speaker, ALM Zone fit leader, Young Living Essential Oils essential oil enthusiast/educator, and published author. In 2013, she was diagnosed with a severe gluten intolerance and since then has spent many hours creating easy, practical and delicious gluten-free recipes that can be enjoyed by both those who are affected by gluten and those who are not.

Growing up, Hope spent many hours in the kitchen with her Meme (grandmother), and her love for cooking grew from there. While working on her master's degree when her daughter was young, Hope turned to her slow cookers for some salvation and sanity. It was from there she began truly experimenting with recipes and quickly learned she had the ability to get a little more creative in the kitchen and develop her own recipes.

In 2010, Hope started her blog, *A Busy Mom's Slow Cooker Adventures*, to simply share the recipes she was making with her family and friends. She never imagined people all over the world would begin visiting her page and sharing her recipes with others as well. In 2013, Hope self-published her first cookbook, *Slow Cooker Recipes 10 Ingredients or Less and Gluten-Free*, and then later wrote *The Gluten-Free Slow Cooker*.

Hope became the new brand ambassador and author of Fix-It and Forget-It in mid-2016. Since then, she has brought her excitement and creativeness to the Fix-It and Forget-It brand. Through Fix-It and Forget-It, she has written many books, including *Fix-It and Forget-It Healthy Slow Cooker Cookbook*, *Fix-It and Forget-It Favorite Slow Cooker Recipes for Mom*, *Fix-It and Forget-It Favorite Slow Cooker Recipes for Dad*, *Fix-It and Forget-It Cooking for Two*, *Fix-It and Forget-It Crowd Pleasers for the American Summer*, and *Fix-It and Forget-It Slow Cooker Dump Dinners and Dump Desserts*, *Welcome Home Diabetic Cookbook*, and *Fix-It and Forget-It Instant Pot Cookbook*.

Hope lives in the city of Clinton Township, Michigan, near Metro Detroit. She's been a native of Michigan her whole life. She has been happily married to her husband and best friend, Justin, since 2008. Together they have two children, Ella and Gavin, who are her motivation, inspiration, and heart. In her spare time, Hope enjoys traveling, singing, cooking, reading books, spending time with friends and family, and relaxing.